T0195301

THE MOREHOUSE MODEL

THE MOREHOUSE MODEL

How One School of Medicine Revolutionized Community Engagement and Health Equity

RONALD L. BRAITHWAITE, PhD
TABIA HENRY AKINTOBI, PhD, MPH
DANIEL S. BLUMENTHAL, MD, MPH
W. MARY LANGLEY, PhD, MPH
Foreword by Valerie Montgomery Rice, MD

JOHNS HOPKINS UNIVERSITY PRESS | *Baltimore*

© 2020 Johns Hopkins University Press
All rights reserved. Published 2020
Printed in the United States of America on acid-free paper
9 8 7 6 5 4 3 2 1

Cataloging-in-Publication Data is available from the Library of Congress.

Johns Hopkins University Press
2715 North Charles Street
Baltimore, Maryland 21218-4363
www.press.jhu.edu

A catalog record for this book is available from the British Library.

ISBN-13: 978-1-4214-3804-7 (hardcover)
ISBN-13: 978-1-4214-3805-4 (ebook)

Special discounts are available for bulk purchases of this book. For more information, please contact Special Sales at specialsales@press.jhu.edu.

Johns Hopkins University Press uses environmentally friendly book materials, including recycled text paper that is composed of at least 30 percent post-consumer waste, whenever possible.

CONTENTS

We dedicate *The Morehouse Model* to our friend, colleague, and coauthor, Daniel S. Blumenthal, MD, MPH. Dr. Blumenthal was a key member of the research team that conceptualized, planned, and authored this volume from the Alpha to the Omega. He met his untimely death on July 25, 2019. He contributed meaningfully by offering his expertise in and to every aspect of the book and served as the institutional memory for many of its components. Without his participation, *The Morehouse Model* would never have come to fruition. He was the most senior of the four coauthors, and, in many ways, he mentored each one of them.

Dr. Blumenthal graduated from Oberlin College in Oberlin, Ohio, in 1964 with a degree in zoology. In 1968, he was awarded his medical degree from the University of Chicago. In 1986, he received his master of public health from Emory University. His career started as a VISTA volunteer in Marianna, Arkansas. He later became an Epidemic Intelligence Service officer at the Centers for Disease Control and Prevention in Atlanta, Georgia.

Over his career, he served as principal investigator for more than 70 grants that generated $60 million; he published over 100 book chapters and journal articles and authored or coedited five books. He rose through the academic ranks to full professor in and chair of the Department of Community Health and Preventive Medicine and held that position for 30 years. From 1991 to 1992, he did a sabbatical at the World Health Organization in Geneva, Switzerland. He also served as a chief health officer for the Fulton County Health Department. For over 20 years he served as the associate dean for community health at Morehouse School of Medicine.

His education, clinical, and public health leadership was extraordinary, and his dedication to service to both Morehouse School of Medicine

(MSM) and the broader disciplines of community-engaged public health and prevention was a class act. He was elected to the presidency of the Association of Teachers of Preventive Medicine, where he served with distinction. He also served as the president of the American College of Preventive Medicine. Dr. Blumenthal retired from Morehouse School of Medicine as Department of Community Health and Preventive Medicine professor and chair emeritus in 2014. Although he was retired, he was frequently on campus guiding and mentoring students, staff, and faculty, across tenure levels, in the art and science of prevention. Dr. Blumenthal was appointed Extraordinary Professor of Community Health from Stellenbosch University Faculty of Medicine and Health Science in Cape Town, South Africa. He was the founding director and principal investigator for the Centers for Disease Control and Prevention–funded MSM Prevention Research Center, where he proudly maintained a senior consultant role until his passing.

Awards received during his career include the Sellers-McCroan Award, Georgia Public Health Association, 1994; the Outstanding VISTA Volunteer of the 1960s (Recognition at the 30th Anniversary Celebration, 1995); the Shining Light Award, Georgia Association for Primary Health Care, 2005; the Leonard Tow Humanism in Medicine Award, MSM, 2005; the Distinguished Alumni Achievement Award, Emory University Rollins School of Public Health, 2009; and the Duncan Clark Award, Association for Prevention Teaching and Research, 2010.

Dan's leadership and unwavering commitment to and support of social justice issues were entrenched in his contributions to community-focused research, clinical practice, education, and service. They are unparalleled. He understood how White privilege operated and that Black lives matter, long before the term and movement were formally advanced. Until the day of his passing, his passion to advance community-engaged leadership (locally, nationally, and globally) was witnessed and felt by not only his *The Morehouse Model* coauthors but also his collaborators, mentees, students, and close friends, nationally and globally.

Given the above resume of professional service, Dan's life work was evidence of the impact he made in the hundreds of careers that he launched among junior faculty and lay citizens in Georgia communities and throughout the world. Dr. Blumenthal's legacy will be commemorated yearly at the Annual Daniel S. Blumenthal Health Conference and Public Health Summit at Morehouse School of Medicine.

Ronald L. Braithwaite
Tabia Henry Akintobi
W. Mary Langley

Valerie Montgomery Rice, MD
President and Dean, Morehouse School of Medicine

This volume seeks to document the legacy that Morehouse School of Medicine (MSM) faculty, staff, and community partners have established, maintained, and scaled as community engagement thought and action leaders for health equity. This work has spanned over 40 years. This book highlights significant community engagement contributions aligned with the MSM institutional mission and designed to reduce and eventually eliminate local, national, and global racial and ethnic health disparities.

MSM was founded in 1975 in Atlanta, Georgia, just after the civil rights era, when color barriers prevented racial minorities from receiving adequate health care and Black students were underrepresented in predominantly White medical schools. MSM was conceived to address both issues as a minority-serving institution educating doctors destined to practice in underserved communities.

Metropolitan Atlanta has the widest gap in breast cancer mortality rates between Black women and White women of any US city and the nation's highest death rate for Black men with prostate cancer. Large gaps in mortality exist between Blacks and Whites in HIV, stroke, diabetes, and other major causes of death, both in Georgia and nationally. Moreover, periodic health needs assessments conducted by the authors of this book in communities served by MSM indicate that major health concerns in the community include high blood pressure, diabetes, overweight, and sexually transmitted infections.

The MSM mission and history continue to be dedicated to changing the health landscape for inner-city and rural communities, while resolving the historical chasm between communities and the academy. This audacious undertaking has been largely achieved in collaborating communities by earning the trust of community partners and positioning them as senior partners rather than solely participants. These efforts are intrinsically aligned with the MSM mission statement, which affirms that we exist to

- improve the health and well-being of individuals and communities;
- increase the diversity of the health professional and scientific workforce; and
- address primary health care through programs in education, research, and service with emphasis on people of color and the underserved urban and rural populations in Georgia, the nation, and the world.

MSM is one of four historically Black medical schools in the United States. Among all the medical schools in the United States, MSM is distinguished by its national leadership in primary care and sustained outreach to disenfranchised populations. As noted in chapters 3 and 4, the school has been recognized repeatedly at both the local and the national level for its community-oriented initiatives in teaching, research, patient care, and service.

MSM was founded by visionaries with a passionate commitment to "serve the underserved." Over its 40-year history, MSM has established a strong relationship and bond of trust with minority communities. MSM has achieved national stature based on its trailblazing focus on community outreach and primary care delivery programs to high health disparity neighborhoods. It is recognized that academic health centers that have earned the trust of underserved communities are in a unique position to provide scientific leadership that advances the health status of populations of color. Unfortunately, far too many majority universities give "lip service" to health equity issues, without the full institutional commitment. The work documented in this book shines light on a model of genuine and sustained citizen participation in collaborative planning, execution, evaluation, and dissemination.

The authors of this volume are not "helicopter researchers," who fly into communities, collect data, and abscond to publish papers. Instead, like the majority of the MSM faculty, they are passionately committed to working collaboratively with communities in a participatory manner. As reported by Mullan, Chen, Petterson, Kolsky, and Spagnola in the *Annals* *of Internal Medicine,* * MSM is the leading medical school in the nation in the area of social mission among the 140 US osteopathic and allopathic medical schools. The authors recognize that addressing social determinants of health is fundamental to combating the daunting health and medical issues among disenfranchised communities. Braithwaite, Akintobi, Blumenthal, and Langley have organized community coalitions for health promotion and disease prevention issues, collectively, for over 130 years. These coalitions have often gone on to address broader social issues. For instance, in a low-income predominantly Black community in southeast Atlanta, the coalition developed to oversee the MSM Prevention Research Center worked with others to prevent the siting of a junkyard, to advocate successfully for the rezoning of an industrial area, to redevelop blighted housing, and to replace a low-end liquor store with a small, attractive shopping center. In another example, for decades, MSM's Health Promotion Resource Center has organized coalitions in rural southwest Georgia to combat drug abuse among Black teens, and these coalitions have also addressed other youth risk factors. In yet another example, they partnered with the Atlanta Housing Authority in three west Atlanta neighborhoods on a federal grant that coordinates health care for 7,200 community residents, connects 850 to medical homes, and secures health insurance for 600. Students provide approximately 9,000 annual community service hours to the project. These examples are areas where faculty have reached hard to reach the hard-to-reach.

The authors and other faculty have also been intentional in their efforts to train, equip, and empower community residents to lead or equitably collaborate in research, policy, and other initiatives they develop to improve communities. The authors of this volume have led the way in developing and collaborating with community health leaders who are educated, motivated, and mobilized to lead and co-labor with community groups in changing health behavior, improving environmental health, and influencing policies to support community health and equity.

---

*Mullan, F., C. Chen, S. Petterson, G. Kolsky, and M. Spagnola. 2010. "The Social Mission of Medical Education: Ranking the Schools." *Annals of Internal Medicine* 152 (12): 804–11. doi:10.7326/0003-4819-152-12-201006150-00009. Erratum in: *Annals of Internal Medicine* 153 (3): 212.

Since its inception, Morehouse School of Medicine (MSM) has been growing social capital. It is a formidable institution committed to community engagement with an interest in closing the health equity gap between people of color and White or majority populations. Being recognized repeatedly for the social mission goal of reaching hard-to-access urban and rural at-risk citizens has become part of the school's DNA. Using a "boots on the ground" approach, community health promotion and disease prevention have brought substantial change to the citizens of Georgia. Moreover, these efforts have affected the lives of consumers in both the South and other regions of the United States. This book captures the historical and contemporary essence of enrolling consumers, neighborhoods, and communities into a health problem–solving process designed to improve the quality of life among disenfranchised groups.

In chapter 1, "Introduction to the Morehouse School of Medicine Model," we describe the philosophical, cultural, and contextual grounding of the Morehouse Model. The chapter ends with a description of work with one of our initial communities (Joyland/High Point), where we beta-tested many of our original concepts of community empowerment for health promotion. In chapter 2, "Social Accountability, Medical Education, and Public Health," we drill down on more concrete examples and depictions of the Morehouse Model and give attention to its relationship to social accountability, medical education, and public health. This chapter begins by defining the concept of social accountability in medical education. Drawing on the scholarship from several international organizations, we capture the national and worldwide standards related to the context of accountability in medical education. Reference to World Health Organization documents, the Beyond Flexner Alliance study and the Institute of Medicine's landmark study, *Unequal*

Treatment: Confronting Racial and Ethnic Disparities in Healthcare, will serve as important benchmarks for discussing health standards. Chapter 2 also includes an ethics-based discussion of the responsibility to the public of medical schools that are largely supported by public funds. Attention also is given to how historically Black medical schools contribute to the pipeline issues of training health professionals and how these institutions have uniquely addressed many of the health disparity concerns of the nation. Case studies of model MSM programs are noted to highlight innovative approaches to social accountability in medicine and public health.

In chapter 3, "Community-Based Participatory Research," we expound on the art, science, and practice of conducting a citizen-involved approach to collaborations in research through the work of our Prevention Research Center and its Community Coalition Board, which has been the driving force for catalytic public health prevention and action for over 20 years. The CBPR approach is detailed through other exemplars of community-academic partnerships advancing translation to transformation for community health and health promotion. This chapter details how these partnerships are fostered, deployed, and sustained despite ambivalent resource-funding environments. Attention is also given to the importance of culturally appropriate and evidence-based interventions in enhancing translation of research outcomes to impact policy formation and adoption. In chapter 4, "Evolution of the Morehouse Model for Community Engagement," we discuss the history of programmatic applications, using community coalitions as the central force for moving the health equity needle. The chapter ends with several new additions of concern to Morehouse Model implementers, with an emphasis on voter rights and registration, participatory budgeting, job creation, and social justice as important coalition activities. In chapter 5, "Engaging Micropolitan and Rural Communities in Health Promotion and Disease Prevention," we discuss our experiences in working with many of the 159 counties in Georgia through the Health Promotion Resource Center. Three case studies are presented to depict the dynamics of working with rural and micropolitan areas.

Chapter 6, "Educational and Leadership Development—for Communities, by Communities," addresses institutions' role in community-focused education, leadership development, training, and technical assistance. The strategic engagement of community health workers from priority communities and the curricula employed to train neighborhood residents, clinicians, practitioners, and learners are highlighted. We discuss in detail the frequently underemphasized significance of the training and deployment of systematically prepared faculty, students, and staff steeped in sound community engagement practice through MSM's degree-granting programs. Community leadership programs are also described, including those fundamental to the missions of centers and institutes such as the Satcher Health Leadership Institute and Community Voices. Finally, the institutions' strategically deployed pipeline programs, providing science, technology, engineering, arts, and mathematics exposure and mentoring opportunities for students from underrepresented and underserved communities (from elementary through post-undergraduate levels), are detailed. The examples described in this chapter demonstrate the ways in which MSM strategically develops and promotes well-equipped leaders who lead strategies that catalyze improved population health, as a cross-cutting institutional priority.

In chapter 7, "The Medical School of Tomorrow," we offer a futuristic perspective based on the Morehouse Model—what the medical school of the future should ideally look like. Medical education is changing from the model prescribed in 1912 by Abraham Flexner to one that features integrated curricula, educational technology, and a heightened focus on the community. Schools founded since 1975— of which MSM is one—emphasize education and community engagement over laboratory research. Much of the education takes place at sites far from the central campus and tertiary care hospitals. This chapter explores the trajectory these trends are likely to take during the next few decades as many medical schools focus far more of their research on the community and on primary care and offer service that goes beyond specialty medical care. These schools strive to graduate a new kind of doctor—one who is prepared to care for his or her community, as well as the patients seen, one at a time in the office or clinic.

In the appendixes we make available to readers the numerous resources deployed by the MSM collective to implement CBPR programs across both urban and rural communities. The tools and instruments referenced include community needs assessment protocols, CBPR curriculum and training manuals, technical assistance and workshop formats, evaluation tools, and an annotated bibliography of published works by MSM implementers and investigators.

The authors are greatly appreciative of the support provided by the Department of Community Health and Preventive Medicine (CHPM) at Morehouse School of Medicine in completing this project. Specifically, the clerical support provided by Tascia Smith, Karmen Jordan, and Cicely Reed was essential to bringing the project to fruition. Research support was also provided by Joyce Sheats, a long-time staff member within CHPM. We appreciate the data reduction support provided by Bea Raiford and the library citation support provided by Roland Welmaker Sr. Angela Wimes also played a vital role with her editing assistance.

Special thanks are extended to the following—Carla Durham Walker, Danielle Duvernay, Rita Finley, Christopher Ervin, Natalie Hernandez, Stephanie Miles-Richardson, Folashade Omole, Gail Mattox, Rhonda Holliday, Pricilla Pemu, Desiree Rivers, Rondereo Sidney, Alice Jackson, Jareese K. Stroud, Beverly Deaderick Taylor, Robina Josiah Willock, Latrice Rollins, LaShawn Hoffman, Meryl McNeil, Daphne Byrd, Fred Murphy, Kisha Holden, Robert Mayberry, Kofi Kondwani, Henrie M. Treadwell, Gregory Strayhorn, Rakale Quarells, the Prevention Research Center Community Coalition Board, and Virginia Floyd—for their contributions, either indirectly or directly, toward informing the community engagement content/context associated with the centers, departments, initiatives, or institutes they lead or support or with which they are affiliated. Many thanks to Loren Peabody, research fellow at the Participatory Budgeting Organization, for his research assistance.

Lastly, we express sincere appreciation to Robin W. Coleman and Adelene Jane Medrano at Johns Hopkins University Press. Without Robin's supportive efforts, this book would not have seen the light of day. We also appreciate the great copyediting work by Jeremy Horsefield.

THE MOREHOUSE MODEL

ONE

Introduction to the Morehouse School of Medicine Model

FROM SMALL beginnings, Morehouse School of Medicine (MSM) was born in July 1975 as an appendage to Morehouse College, with the visionary leadership of a doctor originally from Georgia (Louis W. Sullivan) and the president of Morehouse College (Hugh Gloster). Its inaugural mission was to provide education and training to students from minority and disenfranchised groups to increase the primary care workforce for underserved populations in rural and inner-city areas. This mission remains constant today, yet it has morphed into a more robust platform involving health equity, community engagement (CE), public health practice, cutting-edge research, and patient-centered health care. Indeed, over its 45-year history, MSM has become a major player in the training of minority health professionals and the pursuit of health equity. The institutional mission also focuses on a genuine concern for improving the health status of marginalized citizens in Georgia and wherever MSM graduates serve. These graduates have received training that fosters an appreciation for the plight of indigenous persons who typically have little voice in the access and management of their health care.

This book describes MSM's approach to CE. This process has increased citizen participation in planning and implementing health promotion and disease prevention programs. There is both an art and a science to effective CE. One such approach we discuss is the "Morehouse

Model." The Morehouse Model is described and examples offered throughout this volume, and the key elements that constitute the model across the institution's academic units are detailed. Although the leadership in this arena has been disproportionately provided by faculty and staff in the Department of Community Health and Preventive Medicine, virtually every department and center in the school has contributed.

So, how is the Morehouse Model described? What is it? What are the elements and component steps? Is it driven by theory? How do you encapsulate it? The answers to these questions are rooted in the philosophy, cultural context, and practice behavior of faculty at MSM.

Philosophically, recognizing the community and the interests of the community as central and paramount represents a huge paradigm shift for university faculty. Traditionally, faculty have worked in ivory towers, far distant from the community they serve both conceptually and often physically. Working in communities on health empowerment projects thus calls for a new way of thinking and acting. For forward-thinking universities working with communities, this has been a watershed movement. The word "community" has been defined by many dimensions, for instance, geography, common values, socioeconomic status (SES), or health status. One can be part of the homosexual community, which transcends geography and space. One's community could be defined in terms of race, gender, religion, and national origin, and all of these factors give rise to the intersectionality and complexity of defining a community.

The Morehouse Model has at its core the notion of being a consistent and a trusted partner bridging the "town and gown" through collaboration on planned change in health equity. Philosophically, this depicts a Robin Hood approach to the distribution of limited resources inasmuch as the goal is to provide health services to all in the community. Far too many universities pay lip service to CE but never internalize or actualize the true meaning of the concept or philosophy. As a trusted partner, MSM is fully committed to the goal of community first.

Recognition of the *cultural context* is a necessary and essential aspect of the Morehouse Model. To fully understand cultural context, one must consider how culture can affect the behavior of a group or community and think about the learned values and shared attitudes among groups of community members. Hence, language, norms, values, ideas, customs, and belief systems all make up the cultural context.

Consensus is evident in social scientists' definition of cultural appropriateness and relevance. Culture has been traditionally defined to imply an integrated pattern of human behavior that includes thoughts, communications, actions, customs, values, belief systems, social norms, and material traits of racial, ethnic, religious, or social groups. Some older African Americans, for example, believe that having a medical-surgical procedure and allowing organs to be exposed to air will lead to a more serious outcome than not having surgery at all. The Jehovah's Witnesses religious denomination rejects the medical practice of blood transfusions. For them, good health care translates into cultural practice based on a religious belief system. In some subcultures the acquisition of manhood is linked to the act of losing one's virginity. In many cultures in the developing world, polygynous relationships (wherein a man may have more than one wife) are an accepted countrywide norm. In other subcultures, it is typical to apply salt to one's food before ever tasting it. In the US drug culture, a typical practice involves the sharing of paraphernalia and intravenous needles. Traditional Western cultural standards would view all of these behaviors as high risk and inappropriate for healthy living. Such traditional Western perceptions represent only the tip of the iceberg when one considers the insensitivity of mainstream approaches designed to address health promotion interventions across these culturally different value systems.

In light of the foregoing, those who work in the field of health promotion should strongly consider the role that cultural beliefs have in consequent health promotion programming. One must consider the contextual, cultural, and subcultural group-specific data about the target population SES variables; their awareness and attitude toward disease and wellness; their perceptions of what constitutes high-risk behaviors; and their degree of participation in such high-risk behaviors.

Since the Morehouse Model is largely predicated on African American populations, much attention is given to their historical struggle to find solutions to everyday survival issues and their limited access to state-of-the-art health care, including, but not limited to, diminished employment and education opportunities, income inequality, and a host of other SES factors that negatively impact communities of color. African Americans like to engage in fellowship with others through social gatherings. Having a meeting place can be key to convening CE activities where health promotion programs can be infused. An understanding at MSM of the community cultural context bodes well for acceptance of the community as a necessary and essential partner in fulfilling the mission of MSM. The school's success is dependent on embracing the interests and needs of the community, broadly defined.

Regarding *practice*, MSM was founded on principles of reaching out to the poor and to disenfranchised rural and urban populations. Hence, the school's practice mode has been and will continue to be touching and reaching out to underserved populations and providing them with primary care solutions and disease prevention and health promotion strategies. In addition to the programs of the MSM Department of Community Health and Preventive Medicine, the practicum and clerkship activities of the six other clinical departments (Family Medicine, Medicine, Pediatrics, Surgery, Psychiatry, and Obstetrics and Gynecology) all have varied community outreach projects. Other institutes and centers within MSM also offer community-centered programs. These clinical departments make use of full-time physician faculty and adjunct faculty in community settings to assist with training our students and residents. After graduation, these students and residents carry the MSM brand of primary care and a client-centered orientation with them as they practice at the community level throughout the nation.

As early as 1960, schools of social work were among the first to begin advocating for engaging community organizations as a method for community change. They trained professionals to serve as community organizers to facilitate change in health and human services, health policy, and health care practice. Community organizers have in recent years served as community health workers (CHWs), navigators, and *promotoras* (a Spanish term for "community health workers"). Regardless of the titles assigned to these facilitators, they have maintained the same role, bringing consumers to the table and bringing voice to the voiceless. They are often conveners of the CE process. Some of the early giants and advocates for community organizing include Saul Alinsky (the founder of modern community organizing);[1] Cesar Chavez (an American labor leader and civil rights activist who cofounded the National Farm Workers Association in 1962 along with Delores Huerta); John McKnight (Director of the Community Studies Program at the Center for Urban Affairs and Policy Research at Northwestern University), who is nationally recognized for his book *Community Building from the Inside Out: A Path toward Finding and Mobilizing a Community's Assets*);[2] and Paulo Freire, the Brazilian educator and philosopher who was the leading advocate for critical pedagogy and is best known for his work *Pedagogy of the Oppressed*,[3] considered to be one of the foundational texts of the critical pedagogy movement. More contemporary scholars on CE theory and practice—especially community-based participatory research (CBPR)—include Fred Murphy, Nina Wallerstein, Barbara Israel, Meredith Minkler, and Henrie Treadwell.[4, 5, 6, 7]

So, What Exactly Is the Morehouse Model?

When one speaks of a model, we typically picture Venn diagrams, concentric circles, flowcharts, and other abstract graphical depictions of dependent, independent, and interdependent relationships. Linear, bivariate, and multivariate factors are reduced to a pictorial representation to tell a story. Over the 45-year period in which MSM has launched hundreds of CE projects, a unique symbiosis between the academic and community constituents has been created. That said, we are quick to acknowledge that these many projects have had a multiplicity of components, but the majority of them have been grounded in CBPR and/or CE. The vast majority of them have employed CE principles.

The Morehouse Model advances a series of steps for implementing CE at the community level. For clarification, when we speak about CE, we are characterizing a bilateral effort between an academic institution and a community-based organization (CBO), along with participation and partnership with entities from other sectors. The partnership's

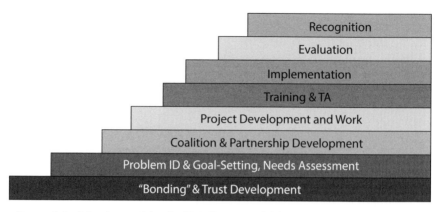

Steps of the Morehouse School of Medicine Model for Community Engagement

initiation and leadership are usually provided by the community and one or more of its CBOs. The agencies, businesses, churches, and other entities are secondary invitees who become an integral part of the whole. Formation of a new coalition partnership is best initiated when the CBO extends an invitation and makes an overture to the academic institution to partner in a joint venture.

Why is the invitation process important to the formation? The invitation is important since many universities doing work in the community are often there to implement their own agenda, or they enter the community to test or implement an intervention that they have developed unilaterally. Far too much faculty-initiated research involving communities is implemented using the helicopter phenomenon, in which the faculty swoops down on a community to collect data and then absconds with the data to publish and write about the community in professional journals. This observation has been well documented over the past 20 years in the CE literature. The approach is antithetical to the Morehouse approach. Hence, the invitation by the CBO establishes a more conducive climate for establishing a genuine, equitable, and balanced collaboration. Equity is critical to any CE effort. Equity in conjunction with a recognition of bilateral learning by both "town and gown" is ideal. Thus, a learning community environment is established from the beginning, which is occasioned by the invitation process.

Step 1. Bonding and Trust Development

A basic and early step in the coalition initiation process is bonding and trust development. A small cluster of three to five persons representing the community and academic institution are often the nucleus driving the process. Having savvy faculty with people skills to link up with CBO persons makes for a new and healthy beginning. Bonding and trust development is an essential and the most important step for sustaining a relationship. In the Morehouse Model, it is step 1 that will allow the two main partners (the academic and the CBO partners) to have a bonded relationship that will fortify the partners against antagonistic forces that will surely emerge during the life of the partnership. This step should not be underestimated in terms of its significance for long-term sustainability. The development of bonding and trust reminds us of the African proverb "If you want to go fast, go alone. If you want to go far, go together." It speaks to the concept of teamwork and mutual respect.

While partners will often disagree and debate many things, maintaining a deep bond and trust will help overcome these obstacles. Hence, bonding and trust allow consensus to be reached when disparate approaches are debated. One does not want to be in a foxhole with a partner fighting an enemy unless bonding and trust have been demonstrated.

Step 2. Problem Identification, Goal Setting, and Needs Assessment

The Morehouse Model makes use of a triangulation approach to problem identification. By triangulation, we simply mean that multiple sources of input are considered when defining the nature of health issues. For example, if we consider the problem of underage drinking, one could listen to the perceptions and accounts of neighborhood residents through surveys, focus groups, and/or key informant interviews. One could collect information from local law enforcement agencies on teen driving under the influence or collect emergency room admissions data on young people involved in accidents due to alcohol consumption. These data can be mapped and analyzed to tell a story about the prevalence of underage drinking along with other data sources (e.g., zip codes). The use of macroagency data, typically in the form of agency annual reports, is often a good starting place for understanding the nature and dynamics of a health challenge present in a community or locale. Problems, challenges, and community concerns are often multifaceted in their manifestation. These issues are not linear and can be assessed by accessing multiple sources. This is true both for problem identification and for a more in-depth community needs assessment.

Needs assessments at MSM have used a variety of analytic methods to document community health issues. Methods such as surveys, interviews, observations, focus groups, asset mapping, geographic information systems (GISs), literature reviews, and secondary analyses of databases have all been employed. Depending on the primary question—be it research, health promotion, or evaluation—the method is driven by the nature of the question. Hence, in the following chapters, cases will be presented that have employed a variety of behavioral and social science methods to document needs in the community.

Once community needs have been documented, typically the Morehouse Model advocates for a priority- and goal-setting process since communities are likely to have numerous issues or concerns. It is essential to set priorities and goals for addressing the most pressing issues. More importantly, as it relates to health issues, it is critical to start with an issue perceived as most important by the community residents. The faculty members and scientists working with the partnership may know from the health science literature that cardiovascular disease is the number one killer in the African American community. If the community is more concerned with substance abuse issues, the Morehouse Model calls for working on the community's priority issue first. Doing this fosters trust and bonding and sets the stage for branching out into future issues such as prevention of heart disease and related cardiovascular health concerns.

Step 3. Coalition and Partnership Development

Numerous national health policy documents published over the past 30 years have called for the involvement of consumers in planning, implementing, and evaluating health-oriented programs. There is an increasing awareness among health planners and health policy makers that the voices of consumers are a critical component of effective health programs. *Healthy People 2000*, *Healthy People 2010*, and *Healthy People 2020* (US health objectives) acknowledge that consumer engagement is an important component of health priority setting.[9, 10] Two reports from the Institute of Medicine (now the National Academy of Medicine)—*The Future of Public Health*[11] and *Unequal Treatment: Confronting Racial and Ethnic Disparities in Health Care*[12]—advocate for local citizen involvement in planning, implementing, and evaluating health-oriented programs. To be clear, these reports are not asking for lay citizens to depart from their lane by serving as clinical planning personnel. Rather, the request to these community consumers is to provide important input for such programs. To have their voices heard is now widely viewed as a value-added element to achieve effective and sustainable health programs in the community.

Among foundations, federal health and human services agencies, voluntary associations, corporations, and private sector philanthropic funding sources, there exists a desire for constituent endorsement and involvement in health and social programming. Never before has a role for constituents been so desirable and demonstrable as a condition of funding. This movement by the numerous funding sources from every sector has been and will continue to be consistent with the CE approach.

Coalition and partnership development is a central part of the Morehouse Model. Throughout this book, coalitions, partnerships, collaborations, and linkage projects are all used interchangeably. The Morehouse Model has given birth to over 75 such coalitions across the 45-year history of MSM. The makeup of these coalitions has varied. All of them have been multisectoral, with community residents being key. These coalitions have often had representation from youth groups, churches and faith entities, CBOs, and macroagencies (education; housing; health;

law enforcement; insurance; parents; business community; media; schools; civic and volunteer organizations; state, local, and tribal government agencies; senior citizens; transportation; recreation agencies; and elected officials). The membership combinations across the coalitions more often than not have been consumer dominated. The size of the coalitions has ranged from 8 to 30 members. Some have become legally incorporated, while others have not. Some subscribe to a Robert's Rules of Order parliamentary structure, while most operate from a consensus decision-making approach. Some of these coalitions have been single-issue while others have been multiple-issue in terms of their aims and emphasis areas. The life cycle for some of these coalitions has been time limited, while others have been ongoing and sustaining entities.

The field has debated the acceptability of establishing time-limited coalitions. The argument in favor of them is typically linked to a funding source that has a beginning and ending, for example, a funded project that seeks to address a temporal issue or a behavior such as car surfing. Once a coalition composed of law enforcement, educators, teens, parents, and so on has been organized to address the dangers of such car surfing behavior and has provided a strong dose of community education about the behavior, then the coalition can dissolve. When the behavior fades and becomes nonexistent in a community or region, the work of the coalition is complete. An argument can be offered for sustaining coalitions when they are not single issue–driven coalitions and there is movement over time to address different community health issues. These coalitions are in for the long haul and include a host of nagging community challenges from substance abuse to unprotected sex to truancy. Of course, many of these issues need to be addressed simultaneously as well.

The initial meetings of the small cluster group will involve discussions about membership and the recruitment of others. Structure and strategic planning will often involve defining group mission and parameters. Some coalitions have employed a Kurt Lewin force-field analysis, some have used a SWOT analysis (strengths, weaknesses, opportunities, and threats), while others have used visioning exercises for defining the scope of the coalition mission, goals, and objectives.[13, 14] The first two approaches are strategic planning tools. The force-field analysis developed in the 1940s by Lewin is a change-management and decision-making tool. The model advances that efforts should be made to transition from conscious wrong to conscious right activities. This is a process and method in which a team or organization begins to predict in advance what the expected resistance will be to a proposed change. Similarly, a SWOT analysis is a tool to be used by a team for making an initial assessment when trying to forecast the lay of the land in an environment. The primary objective of a SWOT analysis is to assist a team, coalition, or organization in developing a more complete awareness of all the factors involved in a decision or plan. Knowing the positive and negative elements in an environment can assist the team in more effectively communicating what parts of a plan need to be recognized by looking at the perceived strengths, weaknesses, threats, and opportunities in the environment.

Step 4. Project Development and Work

The fourth step in the Morehouse Model reinforces the practice of joint and collaborative project development and work. The CBPR principle of involving members in all aspects of an evolving or established partnership is central to the model. When it comes to project development, sometimes the project foci are established on an a priori basis. This is particularly true when a third-party funding source has made a categorical award. With such an award, program planning takes place prior to the grant submission. Project development with a community and an academic institution, when both are committed to CE, begins with the acceptance that both partners have important contributions to make in generating a proposal for submission to a third-party funding source. Following a series of proposal organizing meetings to determine the division of labor and writing assignments, the team needs to reach an early consensus on the goals, objectives, and basic approach. Of course, roles, resources, timelines, budgets, and performance evaluation measures are addressed as well. With the Morehouse Model, planning a community intervention project typically begins with the convening of a few community focus groups on the topic of interest. This helps to ensure relevance and ownership of the resultant project description. Collaborating parties offer input into the conceptualization, design, goal- and objective-setting, implementation strategies, budget preparation, and evaluation processes. Coalition members engage in these same processes when grant funding is not available. The essential ingredient is participatory involvement. The work and skills involved with project development often involve writing and submitting grants for funding.

At MSM, grant writing is a major activity since the school relies on extramural funding to implement many of its programmatic initiatives. This is especially true of those projects that are community-based and community-driven initiatives linked to health equity, health promotion, and disease prevention. These collaborations have a direct impact on changing behaviors and health practices among local consumers. For example, an initiative on food security will be designed to give consumers better access to more and healthier food choices. Thus, the supply chain aspect is important for accessing such healthy foods. Transportation, high-quality grocery outlets, and other social and economic resources become paramount to nutritional intake with urban and rural disenfranchised populations. In later chapters, the dynamics and examples of effective CE strategies employed by Morehouse Model implementers will be detailed, with emphasis on rural and urban populations.

Step 5. Training and Technical Assistance

Through ongoing discussions among coalition team members, ideas and topics in need of more knowledge and training are mentioned and identified. These are the areas in which training and technical assistance needs are expressed and require a resource person with expertise to assist with formally delivering educational input to address the knowledge gap. These needs can also often be identified by simply asking the question, "What are our training needs?" Depending on the training or technical assistance topic, the resource for delivering the training or technical assistance can be identified and recruited from inter-

Table 1.1 Coalition Training and Technical Assistance Topics

Strategic Planning	Dealing with the Media	Interpersonal Communication
Organization Development	Selecting/Developing Health Interventions	Short-Range Planning
Resource Development		Long-Range Planning
Leadership Skills	Substance Abuse Prevention Programs	Program Reporting
Community Problem-Solving	Proposal Development	Program Development
Project Management	Conflict Resolution	Newsletter Development
Fiscal Management	Board Staff Relationships	Community Health Needs Assessment Surveys
Community Organization	Program Evaluation	
Coalition Member Recruitment Strategy	Supervising Staff Personnel	Community Mobilization Strategies
Effective Meeting Management	Team Building	
Communication Skills	Use of Consultants	Nonprofit Incorporation
	Obtaining Technical Assistance	IRS Tax-Exempt Status

nal or external sources. The Morehouse Model relies on training and technical assistance for managers, CHWs, academic faculty, agency personnel, and stakeholders across the partnership and in the community (as both receivers and providers of training and technical assistance). A lesson learned while implementing the model is the observation that training is crucial for capacity development. While coalition meetings have a planned agenda for transacting the management business of the coalition, time is usually set aside at these meetings for discussion and presentation on topical subjects that enable the coalition to grow and fortify new knowledge. Training is usually designed and developed through workshops, seminars, webinars, podcasts, short courses, and so on. It is important to always articulate up front what the training objectives are for a training program. Continuing education units are offered for more structured and advanced trainings.[15] The list of training given in table 1.1 reflects many of the topics addressed across MSM projects.

Step 6. Implementation

Within the Morehouse Model, implementation means applying the prevention, intervention, and policy initiatives designed to deliver, test, and replicate best practices. Implementation seeks to apply science to address health disparity goals. Implementation is also viewed as a bilateral activity with community agencies, CBOs, and academic partners. Typically, the development of a logic model serves as a blueprint for implementation since it identifies all major activities. Role clarification and delineation of tasks by implementers help to keep all players in their lane. Frequent project staff meetings, use of electronic mail, and conference calls are the preferred methods of communication to support the flow of information among members of the partnership team. Effective internal and external communications serve to reduce confusion, misunderstanding, and conflicts among partnership members. The Morehouse Model encourages partners to openly challenge each other to ensure that planned implementation strategies are being delivered with fidelity.

Step 7. Evaluation

Evaluation is a critical step in the Morehouse Model that serves several purposes. Evaluations are often used to address issues of plausibility, probability, and advocacy. For example, plausibility helps us to address concerns about the extent to which an intervention attains expected goals. With a probability assessment, a more robust design is required to determine cause and effect when evaluating the impact of competing approaches. At a lower level of inference, an adequacy assessment is used to merely address whether or not the goals set by the program developers were met. For example, in a global health project on child health that seeks to reduce child mortality to 25 percent in selected villages, an adequacy assessment will attempt to show whether or not this 25 percent target was reached.

Evaluation has developed into a science that relies on behavioral science methods to assess the strengths and weaknesses of program implementation. One of the main questions to be asked when doing an evaluation is, "What difference did it make?" Evaluation is viewed as an ongoing process at the inception of a new program. Formative evaluation is usually done early in the life cycle of a program. For example, for a five-year project, formative evaluation would typically be done during the first 18 months. This evaluation pays close attention to fidelity and the extent to which the project is adhering to the project as planned. Formative evaluation provides feedback to the project managers during the early life cycle of the project and encourages midcourse corrections to ensure fidelity. Use of staff debriefing sessions and booster sessions to monitor implementation helps to ensure congruence of objectives with planned results. Once managers are comfortable with the integrity of the implementation, summative evaluation can be launched. Essentially, the summative approach is usually tied to an annual benchmark or to the end of a project year.

For both formative and summative evaluations, social science analytical tools are used in surveys, interviews, systemic data collection of project performance records, attendance records, and meeting minutes. Evaluation methods are also one of the areas for staff and partner training and technical assistance. Within the framework of the Morehouse Model, multiple partners have a role in conducting evaluations; it is not the sole province of the academic partners. External funding sources would often require an internal or external evaluation. External or third-party evaluations are seen as more objective and unbiased than internal evaluations. These evaluations make use of contracted consultants. Evaluation studies pose questions based on the stated goals and objectives, and a culminating report details and summarizes the findings, with recommendations to the project management leadership team.

Step 8. Recognition

Numerous volunteers are engaged in coalition partnership work. These individuals spend many unpaid hours working on behalf of the community. Burnout by coalition members causes them to lose interest in the work of the coalition; such loss of interest is a predictable occurrence. Offering a small token of appreciation and holding an annual recognition banquet to acknowledge the contributions of the many hours of volunteerism are key components of the Morehouse Model. The simple practice of saying "Thank you" goes a long way toward sustaining and motivating volunteers to stay the course. An awards and recognition banquet amasses a great deal of social capital for the collaborative members of the coalition and their colleagues.

Building the Case for CE

Without question, the health status of inner-city people of color remains unconscionably low when contrasted with that of White Americans. This disparity and observation are not new but illustrated by a historical and linear trend across all categories of the leading causes of disability and death. Thirty-five years ago, Margaret Heckler, secretary of the Department for Health and Human Services, released the *Secretary's Report on the Status of Black and Minority Health*. This national study drew attention to the health disparities between Black and other ethnic minorities and their White counterparts across age groups and disease entities. This report noted an annual 60,000 "excess deaths" among the nation's Black and ethnic minority group populations.[16] Three years later, in 1988, the Centers for Disease Control and Prevention estimated that the annual number of excess deaths among these groups had grown to 75,000. While documentation of health disparities (infant mortality, longevity, and quality of life) between racial/ethnic minorities and Whites predates these reports by 50 years or more, they relit the spark that ignited a national flame focusing attention on health disparities.

The Heckler Report emphasized that the abysmal disparity was an affront both to our ideals and to the ongoing genius of American medicine. The major contributors to the disparity between Black and White death rates were and still are cancer, cardiovascular disease, stroke, diabetes, substance abuse, homicide and accidents, and infant mortality. Since the 1985 report, Blacks and Latinos in particular have manifested a disproportionately high rate of AIDS-related deaths. With this backdrop, the Morehouse Model, along with support from the Kaiser Family Foundation and the W. K. Kellogg Foundation, launched several major intervention initiatives in Atlanta and southern Georgia. Following a plethora of writings by contemporary community organizers and scholarly opinion leaders, a beta test of a community organization model was implemented in an inner-city southwest section of Atlanta known as the Joyland/High Point community.

With funding awarded to MSM from the Kaiser Family Foundation in Menlo Park, California, a CE surveillance approach was advanced and implemented by the Health Promotion Resource Center (HPRC) at MSM. Along with this somewhat open-ended funding came an acknowledgment by Kaiser of the critical importance of learning from and registering the voices of the community consumers as the drivers of any intervention to be planned. Kaiser wanted to connect with the perceived local needs of the consumer constituents before any effort was made to address health disparity interventions at the local level. Moreover, Kaiser program officers were tuned in to the emerging social determinants of health and had connected the dots between health behaviors, access to health, and health outcomes. They recognized that employment, adequate housing, violence prevention, education, food security, access to mental health services, social justice, access to health insurance and recreational outlets, and other resources were essential for achieving health and community empowerment.

In 1989, Braithwaite and Lythcott reported in the *Journal of the American Medical Society*,

> The approach of the Health Promotion Resource Center uses community development to advance community-based health promotion intervention as the change model. An important aspect of this approach facilitates the development of a decision-making community coalition board to identify its health promotion priorities, to inventory its resources, and to build coalitions with the public and private sectors to access other resources and to address policy and manage resources in support of health interventions. This approach also develops community leadership for health promotion and advocates community health promotion. The expectation is that community organization and development for health promotion is a model that will improve the community's ability to address other important quality-of-life issues as well as to improve the health status of its members.

Because health behaviors are culture-bound, primary prevention efforts that address preventable disease and illness must emerge from a knowledge of and a respect for the culture of the target community to ensure that both the community organization and development effort and any interventions that emerge are culturally sensitive and linguistically appropriate. For the poor, such an empowerment approach to health promotion is like a sleeping giant—when it rises up, all will know that the historically disenfranchised will be more self-reliant and healthier.[17]

After identifying a nucleus group of community residents within the Joyland/High Point community, a surveillance strategy sought to organize a household survey using a systematic random sampling design. The thinking between the nucleus group and two HPRC staff community organizers was to attempt to sample a subset of the community heads of household. A sampling frame was generated by listing all of the homes/apartments in Joyland/High Point and then selecting residents of every fourth home/apartment from the list to respond to a household survey designed to acquire information about perceptions of health-related issues in the community. Health in this context was broadly defined to include environment and disease entities. A cadre of community residents and college students were trained on how to administer the household survey during early evenings.

The Empowerment Process

Empowerment represents the undergirding theoretical framework for the Morehouse Model. Freire maintains that an essential component of the empowerment process is that power must be taken from the oppressors by the oppressed, and as a result, the oppressors will be forced to recognize the immorality of their position.[3] This conceptual model may be radical but should not frighten CHWs, especially those who view their roles as community change agents. The Freirian approach has received international acclaim for its contribution to addressing the problem of illiteracy in Brazil. The relationship between quality education and literacy is analogous to the relationship between healthy lifestyle and preventable mortality and morbidity. If disenfranchised populations are able to gain control over one aspect of their lives, this increases the probability that they will be able to gain control over other aspects as well. Empowerment for health promotion provides a framework within which many social ills can be addressed; ultimately, all these ills have an impact on health status. The disenfranchised do not have access to private health clubs, nor, in most cases, do they even have access to culturally and linguistically appropriate health education materials. Braithwaite and Lythcott cited research by Kretzmann and McKnight that suggests that it is impossible to enhance health status among the powerless unless the tools of gaining and exercising authority, such as control of budgets, increased income, and policy decision-making, are transferred to them.[2]

The Joyland/High Point Community

The HPRC at MSM was established to provide training and technical assistance that address primary prevention needs of minority and poor populations. The philosophy of the HPRC is that health promotion efforts are likely to be more successful in these populations when the community at risk is empowered to identify its own problems, develop its own intervention strategies, and form a decision-making coalition board to make policy decisions and manage resources around the interventions. Further, because health and illness behaviors are culture bound, primary prevention efforts to address preventable disease and illness must emerge from a knowledge of and respect for the culture of the target community. This is essential in ensuring that the community organization, development effort, and any health interventions that emerge are culturally sensitive and linguistically appropriate. The HPRC sought to organize and empower minority and poor communities to take an active and participatory role in the identification of their health problems and the planning, design, and implementation of appropriate health promotion programs. In 1988, this work in Joyland/High Point launched the CE approach central in many of the current MSM programs. In an effort to operationalize the community organization and development strategy, several action steps are desirable. These steps are

(1) developing a demographic and epidemiologic profile of the target area, (2) initiating appropriate community entry processes, (3) establishing community trust and credibility, (4) learning the ecological dynamics of the community, (5) organizing a consumer-dominated decision-making community coalition board, (6) facilitating community involvement in the needs assessment process, and (7) further ensuring community ownership through consumer participation in the planning and design of the health promotion intervention. This is achieved by training the community coalition board members to provide them with the tools needed to make policy and resource allocation decisions with regard to the intervention—in other words, teaching them how to fish rather than feeding them fish.

Target Community Profile

The Joyland/High Point community in Atlanta, Georgia, was selected by the HPRC as the community in which to document and analyze the process of community organization. Development criteria included the following factors:

- low-income status, by federal standards;
- a community with high indices of preventable morbidity and mortality;
- a community concerned about one or more lifestyle health risk factors;
- a community with some active indigenous leadership; and
- a community that has not already been organized for health promotion.

Both single- and multifamily residential housing existed within this neighborhood, where approximately one-half of the units are publicly owned or supported. In the early years of the twentieth century, the urban community was an amusement park for Black Atlantans. It included several dance halls, a club, and tracks for horses and bicycles. In 1923, the property was purchased by two real estate developers who designed the present street system and lot lines. Lot sales were slow at first, and it was not until after World War II that significant residential development occurred. Major industry was soon attracted to the area, including a General Motors plant. A US penitentiary was also built in the area. A Black middle-class residential community was established where the amusement park had been, adjacent to the industrial area. However, by 1989, many of the older homes had become dilapidated; newer apartment developments had been constructed specifically for low-income occupancy. According to the 1980 US Census, the Joyland/High Point community had 4,323 Blacks, 34 Whites, and 30 Hispanics. The community had a median household income below $6,500 and a median per capita income below $3,200, with more than 75 percent of the population living at or below the poverty level.[18] Joyland/High Point is located within Neighborhood Planning Unit Y, in southwest Atlanta (with a high incidence of poverty and other ills typical of poverty-stricken areas). Although poverty was widespread, community leaders described their neighborhood with pride and in progressive terms. Some of the single-family homes within the community were well maintained and owned by their occupants. At the time of this work, the only local source of primary health care was a federally funded community health center, which serves adjacent communities as well. According to data collected by the community health center, high blood pressure, asthma, diabetes, acute upper respiratory infection, obesity, homicide, adolescent pregnancy, and substance abuse were the most frequently reported health problems. In addition to the local community health center, the local public hospital was accessible to the community by public transportation.

Guidelines for Community Organization for Health Promotion
Learning the Community

Learning the layout of the community targeted for a health intervention is an essential first step before attempting to enter informal community boundaries.[19] The entry process should begin with a request for geographic and demographic information from local community planning and development agencies. This includes maps that show the basic geography of the target community and block statistical maps that identify census tracts. The Bureau of Census Neighborhoods Statistics Report provides specific statistical summaries essential to determining neighborhood composition. Moreover, identification of neighborhood resources such as schools, hospitals, health centers, police stations, and fire stations was important.

Community Ecology

Learning the community ecology firsthand is essential to the community organization process. This can be achieved by routinely traveling through the community and doing a windshield survey. If the community is large and/or spread out, it will be important to first commute through the community by automobile or the public transportation system. Familiarization with street layout and the daily cycle of human behavior is essential. It is useful to travel through the community during different times of the day (i.e., morning, afternoon, evening). Impromptu visits to the community on weekends and holidays will also provide a different perspective of the community from its weekday ecological rhythm. The CHW should make mental and written notes of where different circles of people gather, where various types of clusters of people converge, and where restaurants, stores, churches, recreation centers, schools, and other community facilities are located. Although using transportation is useful in becoming sensitized to the community, an effective way to learn the community ecology is to walk through the community regularly. In high-risk communities, it is important to be cognizant of personal safety and the community's attitude toward one's presence. In many cases, it is unreasonable to walk through certain areas of the community unless accompanied by a reputable and recognizable community gatekeeper (a formal or informal leader who can provide access to the community).

Prior to entering the community, the CHW must identify and meet with formal and informal gatekeepers of the neighborhood. As the CHW moves through the community and establishes contacts, he or she cannot afford to take anyone for granted. Thus, every encounter and referral to other encounters is to be considered important and should be followed up. Familiarization with names, faces, and places is essential. A daily log serves as a source of recall and documentation for various meetings, names, places, times, and other important information necessary to the organizational process. This documentation is an important way of learning what works in the community organization and development process and what does not. Development of a community resource inventory as a reference source for future planning of the community-based health promotion intervention is also an essential task. It includes names, addresses, and telephone numbers of businesses, churches, schools, health facilities, emergency services, and sources of transportation.

Community Entry Process

It is critical that the entry process be negotiated tactfully with community gatekeepers. Tact is essential in developing trusting, genuine, and nonthreatening relationships. The CHW should exhibit unconditional positive regard and empathy for the local community. Once accepted by the gatekeepers as a community advocate, the CHW will be validated by the formal and informal networks that operate in Black communities. Initially, however, the CHW is likely to be seen as an outsider by residents. Thus, there is a period of suspicion prior to establishing credibility. Making neighborhood contacts, therefore, is an important step toward establishing an identity in the neighborhood and represents an initial opportunity to express a sincere interest in the well-being of the community as a whole. First impressions, in most cases, are lasting ones, and they are essential but not sufficient. True credibility will be assured only through time, commitment, and consistency. One way of identifying important neighborhood leaders, other community gatekeepers, and key community concerns is to contact local elected officials representing the target area. Community health and human service providers are also key sources of information on community contacts, concerns, and barriers to health care. In poor and medically underserved communities, these individuals are extremely helpful in disseminating information about social and health concerns in the community. Business owners, clergy educators, youth workers, senior citizen workers, and other active members of the community are also helpful in accessing smaller circles within the neighborhood.

Building Credibility

Tangible incentives for community participation should be offered. A viable approach to motivating community residents is to assure them that resources and skills are available to facilitate their taking control over their own destiny. The CHW must be able to convince community leaders and brokers of this if progress is to be made in community organizations. After contact with several community leaders, a repetitive theme of community concerns will evolve. The CHW must have a keen ear and identify those problems with which he or she may be able to provide assistance. It is important, however, that one not make a commitment of resources over which he or she lacks control. On the other hand, by providing resources that address community concerns, one can raise the level of community trust.

For example, while organizing in the Joyland/High Point community, an opportunity arose to respond to several community requests to provide a neighborhood football team with jerseys. This represented a small, but important, symbolic gesture of our goodwill. This was an excellent method of beginning to establish credibility. The gesture also may have had a social marketing effect since we requested that the donated jerseys carry a health education message. The team leaders consented, and the jerseys were made with the slogans "Fight Drugs" and "Say No to Drugs." We also coordinated the involvement of several college students as tutors for community youth in a dropout prevention project sponsored by the city of Atlanta. The provision of tutors was another important gesture of goodwill. Establishing rapport and trust is the initial goal of the CHW, but the community need not be asked to give this trust in the absence of genuine advocacy by the CHW.

Development of a Community Coalition Board

The rationale for initiating a consumer-dominated (60% minimum) coalition board is based on social psychology and community organization principles. Such principles acknowledge the benefits of shared decision-making, self-help and self-reliance, and reference group ownership of community concerns, strategies, and approaches to address them.

An early step in the organization of the Joyland/High Point community was initiation of a community coalition board. The board was composed of 18 members, including local consumers and resource persons: the principal of the local high school, an employee of the local recreation center, a local elected official, the pastor of the community church, and one representative each from the Atlanta Junior League, the local community health center, the county health department, and the Atlanta Chamber of Commerce. Thus, the majority of the board members were consumer residents of the Joyland/High Point community.

It is the responsibility of the board to oversee the entire process of community organization and development for health promotion. This includes conducting a community health needs assessment (a door-to-door household survey utilizing trained and paid community interviewers), taking the needs assessment data to the community to facilitate identification of their health priorities, planning and designing the community-based health intervention, and identifying resources (including applying for funds) to support the intervention project. The staff of the HPRC and other MSM faculty were available to provide technical assistance as needed and served as support staff to the community coalition board.

Community Needs Assessment

The community needs assessment in Joyland/High Point was designed to assist the community coalition board and the community in identifying what local residents perceived as their most important health concerns. Asking residents for their input communicates the message that they know what their problems are and that their opinions are important. This helps to promote self-engagement, and the residents are made to feel that their voices can be heard. These benefits are lost, however, unless there is diligent follow-up. For example, respondents in Joyland/High Point were asked whether they would attend a health education workshop. It then became extremely important for us to convene the workshop in order to retain credibility. The strategy used for the Joyland/High Point community needs assessment was to recruit neighborhood residents and a few local college students to serve as household interviewers for the needs assessment survey. These individuals were trained to conduct the interviews and to use the survey instrument. Community interviewers had a pivotal role in the design and refinement of the survey instrument. Again, the genuine involvement of local residents and coalition board members in this important data collection activity signaled to them that we valued their involvement. This method also facilitates ownership by local residents of the data collection methodology, the data itself, and the process of community organization and development for empowerment.

Planning the Intervention

The community coalition board, with the CHW as staff support, should use data collected in the community needs assessment, plus its own knowledge of the community, to identify a health problem or problems to be addressed and to select appropriate health promotion interventions. The CHW should serve as a resource person throughout this process and may even offer a menu of appropriate interventions of demonstrated efficacy that the board may review and revise. However, the community coalition board as representative of the community should retain control and ownership of both the problem identification process and the planning and design of the intervention. When the intervention is initiated, community residents should be employed in every phase of the process.

The CHW should then assist the board in planning implementation of the intervention. This includes facilitating arrangements for board training following an assessment of its training needs. Typical training needs of community coalition boards include problem-solving, board-staff relationships, fiscal management, resource development, grantsmanship, and program evaluation. The CHW may also assist the community coalition board in identifying possible financial resources to support the intervention, such as the local health department, local private sector organizations, national foundations, or the federal government.

Summary

The community organization and development process is not new and has its roots in social action ideology from the 1960s. The difference between the 1960s and the 1990s was in the bringing together of target community consumers with representatives of private and public sector resources (with consumers in the majority) to form a community coalition board. This community coalition board must make policy decisions. The work of CHWs and a mission of health promotion are viable methodologies for addressing the needs of medically underserved and unserved communities. The HPRC at MSM sought to combine the ideology of community organization and development with culturally sensitive and linguistically appropriate health promotion curriculum materials and intervention strategies.

Within this chapter, background information was provided on MSM and its work in health promotion, health equity, and outreach to disenfranchised and underserved urban and rural populations, primarily in Georgia. The Morehouse Model has been described, with attention to the dynamics involved with the eight-step approach to CE. The Morehouse Model has been deployed in many different settings across the clinical departments at MSM; however, it has been primarily used by faculty in the Department of Community Health and Preventive Medicine. An early application and case study of the Joyland/High Point community was our approach to amplify CE. The approach has been evaluated internally and externally across the many health intervention projects where the model was used and found to be impactful.

References

1. Alinsky, Saul D. 1971. *Rules for Radicals*. Toronto: Random House.

2. Kretzmann, John P., and John McKnight. 1993. *Building Communities from the Inside Out: A Path toward Finding and Mobilizing a Community's Assets*. Chicago: Asset-Based Community Development Institute; Northwestern University, Evanston, IL.

3. Friere, Paulo. 1970. *Pedagogy of the Oppressed*. New York: Seabury.

4. Murphy, Frederick. 2012. *Community Engagement, Organizing, and Development for Public Health Practice*. New York: Springer.

5. Blumenthal, Daniel S., Ralph J. DiClemente, Ronald L. Braithwaite, and Selina A. Smith. 2013. *Community-Based Participatory Health Research: Issues, Methods, and Translation to Practice*. New York: Springer.

6. Israel, Barbara A., Eugenia Eng, Amy J. Schulz, and Edith A. Parker, eds. 2012. *Methods for Community-Based Participatory Research for Health*. 2nd ed. San Francisco: Jossey-Bass.

7. Minkler, Meredith, and Nina Wallerstein. 2011. *Community-Based Participatory Research for Health*. San Francisco: Jossey-Bass.

8. Treadwell, Henrie M., Marguerite J. Ro, and Leda M. Pérez. 2010. *Community Voices: Health Matters*. San Francisco: Jossey-Bass.

9. Centers for Disease Control and Prevention and National Center for Health Statistics. *Healthy People 2000, 2010, 2020*. Washington, DC: US Department of Health and Human Services.

10. Institute of Medicine. 2011. *Leading Health Indicators for Healthy People 2020: Letter Report*. Washington, DC: National Academies Press.

11. Institute of Medicine. 1988. *The Future of Public Health*. Washington, DC: National Academies Press.

12. Institute of Medicine Committee on Understanding and Eliminating Racial and Ethnic Disparities in Health Care. 2003. *Unequal Treatment: Confronting Racial and Ethnic Disparities in Health Care*, ed. B. D. Smedley, A. Y. Stith, and A. R. Nelson. Washington, DC: National Academies Press.

13. Lewin, Kurt. 1951. *Field Theory in Social Science*. New York: Harper & Row.

14. Valentin, Erhard K. 2001. "SWOT Analysis from a Resource-Based View." *Journal of Marketing Theory and Practice* 9 (2): 54–69.

15. Braithwaite, Ronald L., Sandra E. Taylor, and John N. Austin. 2000. *Building Health Coalitions in the Black Community*. Thousand Oaks, CA: Sage.

16. US Department of Health and Human Services. 1985. *Report of the Secretary's Task Force Report on Black and Minority Health*. Washington, DC: US Government Printing Office. O-174-719.

17. Braithwaite, Ronald L., and Ngina Lythcott. 1989. "Community Empowerment as a Strategy for Health Promotion for Black and Other Minority Populations." *Journal of the American Medical Society* 261 (2): 282–83. doi:10.1001/jama.1989.03420020136047.

18. US Census Bureau. 1980. *1980 Census*. Washington, DC: US Government Printing Office.

19. Braithwaite, Ronald L., Frederick Murphy, Ngina Lythcott, and Daniel S. Blumenthal. 1989. "Community Organization and Development for Health Promotion within an Urban Black Community: A Conceptual Model." *Health Education* 20 (5): 56–60.

TWO

Social Accountability, Medical Education, and Public Health

What Is Social Accountability?

STARTING IN the late 1990s, a movement developed that advocates for increased "social accountability" in medical education. In more recent years, the movement has gained increased traction and has also acquired alternative labels, such as "social responsibility" and "social mission."

The dictionary definition of "accountability" is "subject to the obligation to report, explain, or justify something; responsible; answerable."[1] "Socially accountable medical education" suggests that medical schools have a responsibility to society to justify their educational programs in return for the support that society provides the schools. The social accountability movement calls on schools to meet the most pressing needs of society rather than pursuing some other set of objectives.

It could be argued that medical schools have no such obligation. American medical students pay tuition for their education. Most of it is borrowed; the average medical student graduates with about $200,000 in educational debt and hence might be seen as accountable only to the bank, not to society. As for the schools (the argument goes), they are supported by these tuition payments, clinical income, and donations and hence have no real responsibility to society at large.

However, tuition income constitutes less than 10 percent of the budget of the typical medical school. Clinical income consists of tax-based payments from Medicare and Medicaid, as well as private insurance. Private insurance is based on premium payments from policyholders—that is, from society. A major portion of the budget of most US medical schools derives from federal grants, especially from the National Institutes of Health (NIH). NIH provided medical schools with more than $13 billion in research grants in 2017.[2] Additional federal agencies that offer grant funding to medical schools include the Centers for Disease Control and Prevention (CDC), the Health Resources and Services Administration (HRSA), the Department of Defense, and others. In addition, medical schools that are part of state universities (over half of all US medical schools) are partially supported by state tax dollars and, as public institutions, have an obligation to the citizens of their state.

Hence, it seems clear that medical schools in the United States should be accountable to the citizenry that supports them through tax dollars and insurance premiums. This is doubly true in most other countries, where medical education is almost wholly financed by taxes, students pay little or no tuition, and, in many cases, faculty conduct little research.

Beyond monetary considerations—and most importantly—physicians and their institutions (medical schools, hospitals, research centers, etc.) are viewed as altruistic entities whose professional ethics obligate them to pursue the best interests of patients, communities, and society. Sometimes this is known as the "social contract" between medicine, medical institutions, and society. Hence, medical schools have a "social mission" that is inherent in the nature of the profession to which they are dedicated.

The social accountability of medical schools was discussed in the medical literature at least as early as 1969.[3] It was defined in a 1995 World Health Organization (WHO) publication as the obligation to direct their education, research, and service activities toward addressing the priority health concerns of the community, region, and/or nation they have a mandate to serve. The priority health concerns are to be identified jointly by governments, health care organizations, health professionals, and the public.[4] That publication contained a "social accountability grid" suggesting that the education, research, and service activities of a medical school be evaluated according to their relevance, quality, cost-effectiveness, and equity.

Very little of the literature on social accountability is the product of American authors. Canada came early to the social accountability table.[5] Medical educators in Canada have generated much of the theoretical framework around "social accountability" and what it means to be a socially accountable medical school,[6,7] and social accountability is now an accreditation criterion for Canadian medical schools.[8] Examples in the literature of socially accountable medical schools and medical education programs have come not only from Canada[9] but also from India,[10] Australia,[11] Uganda,[12] the United Kingdom,[13] and elsewhere.

In the United States, however, there has been some attention paid to the closely related concept of "social mission," and an organization known as the Beyond Flexner Alliance has been developed to focus on this concept.[14] Social mission, as well as the role of Abraham Flexner, is examined in the next section of this chapter.

In the United States, the need for more primary care physicians has been identified as a priority health concern for decades.[15] Similarly, the need for more physicians practicing in rural and inner-city communities has long been an issue.[16] Less discussed, but likewise identified by those who study the medical workforce, is a shortage of physicians specializing in public health and preventive medicine.[17] More recently, racial and ethnic health disparities have been described in the medical literature and in government policy as a priority health concern.[18] While many disease-specific priority health concerns exist, there is widespread agreement that the best way to address them from a health care perspective is through primary care and by providing that care to populations that currently lack it, such as those in rural and inner-city areas.

For Morehouse School of Medicine—a historically Black institution—social accountability includes an explicit intent to address racial and ethnic health disparities and health equity, described in the next section. It also includes a focus on educating more African Americans and other minorities as physicians and biomedical scientists. Minorities are no longer excluded from non-HBCU (historically Black colleges and universities) medical schools as they once were, but they still constitute only a small fraction of the student body at most medical schools. Although African Americans constitute about 13 percent of the US population and Hispanics about 17 percent, they each constitute less than 6 percent of physicians. It has been shown that minority physicians are more likely than White physicians to practice in underserved communities and care for minority patients.[19]

Health Disparities and Health Equity

Racial health disparities first came to public attention in the 1985 government document *Report of the Secretary's Task Force on Black and Minority Health*.[20] Numerous reports, journal articles, books, and conferences ever since have documented persistent disparities in which African Americans have worse health status than any other racial or ethnic group. African Americans have higher mortality rates overall and for every important cause of death (see table 2.1). It stands to reason that a socially accountable medical school will teach about these disparities and develop research and service programs to address them.

More recently, the negative construct of "health disparities" has been turned to the reverse side of the same coin: striving for the positive construct of "health equity." In addition, "health equity" more accurately describes the desired state. A disparity is simply a difference, and not

Table 2.1 Life Expectancy, Age-Adjusted Mortality, and Years of Potential Life Lost by Race and Ethnicity, United States, 2015

Health status	Black	White	Hispanic	Native American[a]	Asian/Pacific Islander
Life expectancy[b]	75.5	79.0	82.0	NA	NA
All cause mortality rate[c]	851.9	735.0	525.3	596.9	394.8
Heart disease[c]	205.1	167.9	116.9	118.5	86.5
Cancer[c]	180.1	159.4	110.3	107.9	99.0
Stroke[c]	50.8	36.4	32.3	24.7	29.8
Unintentional injury[c]	36.8	46.0	28.6	50.7	16.1
Homicide[c]	19.8	3.3	4.9	6.2	1.6
Diabetes[c]	37.0	19.6	25.2	34.2	15.7
HIV infection[c]	7.9	1.1	1.8	1.4	0.4
Influenza and pneumonia	15.9	15.2	11.4	12.5	14.0
Infant mortality[d]	10.7	4.9	5.0	7.6	3.9

Source: Chart courtesy of Dr. Sonja Hutchins, Morehouse School of Medicine.
[a] Native American is the same population as American Indian/Alaska Native.
[b] Life expectancy from birth (in years).
[c] Age-adjusted mortality (deaths per 100,000 population). Available at https://www.cdc.gov/nchs/data/hus/2016/018.pdf. Unintentional injury deaths include opioid overdose deaths.
[d] Infant deaths per 1,000 live births in 2014.

all differences are inequitable. The elderly will, on average, be less healthy than the young; smokers will generally be less healthy than non-smokers. The former is biological and immutable; the second is remediable but is not viewed as unfair. But unlike smoking, race cannot be changed. "Health equity" says that racial disparities are unfair and should be eliminated. MSM has adopted the vision "Leading the creation and advancement of health equity."

Measuring Social Accountability

The WHO approach to assessing the social accountability of medical schools was elaborated in a "global consensus" document developed through a Delphi process by an international reference group (130 organizations and individuals) and finalized by a 20-member steering committee at a meeting in Port Elizabeth, South Africa, in 2010.[21] The document extends the definition of social accountability as a set of challenges: improving quality, equity, relevance, and effectiveness in health care delivery; reducing the mismatch with societal priorities; redefining roles of health professionals; and providing evidence of the impact on people's health status. It offers 43 criteria by which social accountability could be assessed, grouped into 10 thematic areas:

1. Anticipating society's health needs
2. Partnering with the health system and other stakeholders
3. Adapting to the evolving roles of all health practitioners
4. Fostering outcome-based education
5. Creating responsive and responsible governance of the medical and health sciences faculty
6. Refining the scope of standards for education, research, and service
7. Supporting continuous quality improvement in education, research, and service delivery
8. Establishing mandated mechanisms for accreditation
9. Balancing global principles with context specificity
10. Defining the role of society

A document developed nearly simultaneously by an organization known as the Training for Health Equity Network (THENet)[22] offers an evaluation framework.[23] The document is intended as a practical tool for evaluating the level of an institution's social accountability. It does not offer a new definition of social accountability but does offer a set of 10 principles, stating that at socially accountable medical schools

1. health and social needs of targeted communities guide education, research, and service programs;
2. social accountability is demonstrated in action through a "whole school" approach;
3. students are recruited from the communities with the greatest health care needs;
4. programs are located within or in close proximity to the communities they serve;
5. health professions education is embedded in the health system and takes place in the community and clinics instead of predominantly in university and hospital settings;
6. curriculum integrates basic and clinical sciences with population health and social sciences, and early clinical contact increases the relevance and value of theoretical learning information technology;
7. pedagogic methods are student centered, problem and service based, and supported by information technology;
8. community-based practitioners are recruited and trained as teachers and mentors;
9. health system actors are partners to produce locally relevant competencies; and
10. faculty and programs emphasize and model commitment to public service.

It also cites a set of values: relevance, quality, effectiveness, equity, and partnerships. With the addition of "partnerships," these values reflect the elements listed in the 1995 WHO publication. The framework itself is an 11-page matrix listing 14 criteria grouped in three sections ("key components"), with numerous suggested sources of documentation and evidence for each criterion.

Utilizing the framework as an evaluation tool is a substantial undertaking that might be compared in complexity to the preparation of a self-study for accreditation by the Liaison Committee for Medical Education (the accrediting body for medical schools in the United States). However, five schools in Canada, Australia, and the Philippines, supported by foundation grants, piloted evaluation exercises based on the framework and concluded that it "is a practical and useful tool, and [provides a] whole school reflective process for health professional schools to assess their progress toward social accountability."[24, 25]

The Association for Medical Education in Europe developed an awards program called ASPIRE to Excellence.[26] Awards are given annually to medical, dental, and veterinary schools in six areas, one of which is social accountability. The criteria for the social accountability award are derived largely from the *Global Consensus* document. They are listed in four areas:

1. Organization and function, which states that "social accountability is a prime directive in the school's purpose and mandate and is integrated in its day-to-day management."
2. Education of doctors, dentists, and veterinary practitioners, including admissions, curriculum, faculty development, and continuing professional education.
3. Research, which states that "community/regional/national health needs inspire the school's research including knowledge translation."
4. Contribution to health services and health service partnerships for community/region, including partnerships with communities, health care organizations, health managers, policy makers, and government.

Another approach to evaluating social accountability (but using the term "social mission") was developed at Georgetown University and described in 2010 by Mullan et al.[27] This methodology was based on three measures: the percentage of a school's graduates that entered primary care fields, the percentage that practiced in medically underserved areas, and the percentage who were members of minority populations underrepresented in medicine (as compared to their representation in the population at large). This approach is unique in that it utilizes outcome measures to evaluate the extent to which a school has achieved its social mission rather than the process measures (actions the school is taking) proposed by others. The authors ranked the 141 (at that time) US allopathic and osteopathic medical schools. MSM was ranked number one. In a subsequent study, named "Beyond Flexner," they investigated some of the top-ranked schools (plus some newer schools) to explore factors that contributed to their high rankings.

Who Was Flexner?

Abraham Flexner was an educator who, in 1908, was engaged by the Carnegie Foundation for the Advancement of Education to produce a report on medical education in the United States. At the time, the quality of US medical schools was uneven, to say the least. While some schools, such as Johns Hopkins University, provided a rigorous medical education, others offered little more than apprenticeships. Most were somewhere in between those extremes.

Flexner admired the Hopkins model, which in turn was patterned after medical education in European medical schools. His report, published in 1910, recommended that all medical schools should emulate the Hopkins/European curriculum: a college degree should be required for admission, and the medical curriculum should consist of two years of basic science study followed by two years of clinical training in the hospital. Over the next several years, these recommendations were adopted by state regulators, and those schools whose curriculum did not reflect the Hopkins/European model either moved to that model or closed.

Although some medical education reform was underway even before the Flexner Report was published, Flexner is generally recognized as the father of the standard medical curriculum that changed little in the next 70 years. The name "Beyond Flexner" suggests that medical education in the twenty-first century should advance "beyond" that curriculum.

We consider Abraham Flexner and his impact on medical education in more depth in chapter 7.

The Beyond Flexner study used eight modalities[28] and described approaches at exemplary schools—what might be called "best practices" (although the investigators did not use that term):

1. Mission
2. Pipeline
3. Admissions
4. Curriculum
5. Location of Clinical Experience
6. Tuition Management
7. Mentoring
8. Postgraduate Engagement

More recently, the same team developed a Social Mission Metrics Initiative[29] that has compiled a list of 18 areas by which a school can do a self-assessment.

Pursuing Social Mission and Achieving Social Accountability at Morehouse School of Medicine

The Mullan ranking was not the first time that Morehouse was acknowledged for accomplishments that could be termed "social accountability" or "social mission." Recognitions include the Community Service Award from the Association of American Medical Colleges (1999); the First Annual Award from Community-Campus Partnerships for Health, a national organization promoting community engagement by health professions schools (2002); the CDC Outstanding Community-Based Participatory Research Award (2004) and Excellence in Community-Based Research Award (2005); the Carnegie Foundation Classification for Community Engagement (2008); the Georgia Healthcare Foundation Joseph D. Greene Community Service Award (2010); two CDC awards for outstanding community-based participatory research (2010 and 2011); and the Josiah Macy Jr. Foundation Award for Institutional Excellence in Social Mission (2016).

However, the "Beyond Flexner" modalities that derived from the ranking study provide a useful and convenient rubric for describing the approaches that MSM has taken to achieve its success in social accountability and social mission. As indicated above, the same team has now moved to 18 criteria for doing a self-assessment, but, for our purposes, the eight modalities are sufficient.

Mission

The typical medical school mission statement is quite general, for instance, "To lead [state] and the nation to better health through excellence in biomedical education, discovery, patient care, and service." Hence, one might think that mission statements have little real bearing on a school's educational program. However, the social mission content of a school's mission statement has been found to be a strong predictor of the percent of graduates entering family medicine, as well as the percent of graduates working in medically underserved areas.[30]

The MSM mission statement is fairly specific and calls on the school to graduate primary care physicians from underrepresented minority groups who will practice in medically underserved communities. It has been rewritten several times since the school's founding in 1975 but always includes those elements. Its current iteration is as follows: "We exist to improve the health and well-being of individuals and communities, increase the diversity of the health professional and scientific workforce, and address primary health care through programs in education, research, and service, with emphasis on people of color and the underserved urban and rural populations in Georgia, the nation, and the world."

Students, faculty, and staff are all familiar with the mission, and most are able to state it, if not verbatim, at least with respect to the essential elements. It is referenced often in the school's written documents and online content. The school measures its success by the percentage of its students who are minorities and the percentage of its graduates who go into primary care and/or who practice in underserved communities. It is the mission that drives the planning and implementation of MSM's programs.

Pipeline

The rate-limiting factor in recruiting underrepresented minorities into medical education is the size of the minority applicant pool. Building the applicant pool is particularly important for MSM because competition is fierce among medical schools for underrepresented minority applicants with outstanding college grade point averages and Medical College Admission Test (MCAT) scores. Creating an effective "pipeline" means reaching all the way down to elementary school and helping to strengthen children's education, developing their interest in health professions careers, and counseling them on pursuing those careers. MSM supports numerous pipeline programs, such as educational STEAM (science, technology, engineering, arts, and math) academies on Saturdays and during the summer for children in grades K–12. In addition, the school sponsors campus visit opportunities to stimulate interest in medical school among children and adolescents, mentoring programs for K–12 students, summer research programs for high school students, a partnership with an elementary school, and a community health worker training program for high school students.

Since 1984, MSM has offered an Area Health Education Centers (AHEC) program, which is a partially federally funded pipeline initiative that reaches out to minority K–12 and college students, including those from underserved communities, to stimulate interest in health professions careers. AHEC then continues the pipeline by supporting education and training of medical and other health professions students in underserved (particularly rural) communities by offering student housing, orientation, travel reimbursement, and other services. It completes the pipeline by providing continuing education, library services, and other supports to health professionals practicing in underserved communities. As of 2018, the MSM AHEC Program has been merged into the Georgia Statewide AHEC Program conducted by Augusta University/Medical College of Georgia.

Admissions

It is often said that the career trajectory of medical students is already determined when they enter medical school and isn't changed much by the curriculum or any other steps the school may take. If the school wants to graduate more primary care physicians, it is the responsibility of the admissions committee to identify those applicants who are predisposed in that direction. It must be added that this is a bit of "common wisdom" and there are other such bits that are at variance with this one. It does seem likely, however, that selecting students whose values are consistent with those of the school will result in graduates who reflect those values.

Hence, the MSM Admissions Committee bears responsibility, to the extent possible, for identifying applicants who resonate with the idea of becoming primary care physicians practicing in medically underserved communities. It does this by assigning significant weight to "noncognitive" factors in admissions decisions. "Cognitive" factors, of course, include MCAT scores and college grades, the latter weighted by considerations such as the difficulty of courses taken and the need to hold a job while attending college. Noncognitive factors include experiences such as working in homeless shelters, participating in foreign mission trips, and rural origins. Other noncognitive factors include character, responsibility, maturity, compassion, and—of course—an expressed interest in a career in primary care in an underserved community.

These noncognitive factors can be discerned by Admissions Committee members through a careful reading of the personal statement that each applicant must submit as part of the application process and by the applicants' statement and demeanor in an interview. Of course, applicants who are familiar with the MSM mission may claim career intentions that they don't actually feel, and Admissions Committee members must learn to detect clues that will help identify such masquerades. The personal essay is helpful in this regard, since all US medical school applications are submitted through the American Medical College Application Service provided by the Association of American Medical Colleges (AAMC). Each applicant submits a single personal statement that is included in the package that is sent to every school to which the individual is applying. Hence, it is not possible to "tailor" the statement to the priorities of a particular school.

On the matriculation questionnaire at MSM, about two-thirds of students indicate an intent to pursue a primary care specialty and over half plan a career in an underserved area, compared to 35 and 25 percent, respectively, nationally. The mean MCAT scores of entering classes are usually about a standard deviation below that of the national cohort, but on the United States Medical Licensing Examination, Step 1, the class means and pass rates are at or above the national means (on time in two years and with less than 2% attrition; 2015 data).

At MSM, this academic success is usually attributed to the support and attention given to students—particularly those who encounter academic difficulty. In any case, it demonstrates that medical school admissions need not be based solely, or almost so, on college grades and MCAT scores. Other qualities that are important in identifying compassionate, social mission–oriented students can be given major weight, and the final product—the practicing physician—can be just as technically excellent, or more so, compared to the more traditional medical student.

It must be noted that, on average, MCAT scores of racial and ethnic minorities are lower than those of Whites, and that furthermore—as previously mentioned—there is great competition among all medical schools for minority students with outstanding MCAT scores and grade point averages. This competition usually manifests itself in the form of scholarship offers, offers that MSM may have difficulty matching. Hence, in order to build a class comprising 80–90 percent underrepresented minority students, MSM admits many students who have not been accepted at any other school. MSM's ability to develop these students into excellent physicians is the quality that enables the school to "increase the diversity of the health professional and scientific workforce," as called for by the school's mission statement.

Curriculum

As noted earlier, the extent to which a medical school curriculum can influence a student's career choice is controversial. Some medical schools have special primary care tracks, or rural tracks, designed in part to motivate students in the track to choose a primary care (or rural) career.[31, 32] But it is likely that students who enter a rural or primary care track are already inclined to pursue a career in rural medicine or primary care. Perhaps one should consider that a rural or primary care track attracts students interested in a rural or primary care career and the track curriculum reinforces that interest and prepares the student for that career.

However, in discussing curriculum, one must take note of the "hidden curriculum" that exists at most schools of medicine. This refers to the role modeling influence of the specialists and subspecialists who are often the most respected and most renowned (and highest-paid) faculty members. This role modeling is generally thought to be an important factor in influencing students away from primary care, as well as a factor in reducing the humanism and altruism with which most medical students begin their professional education.[33] While the hidden curriculum is, for the most part, hidden—that is to say, implicit and subtle—it is a medical education truism that many of the most outstanding students are told, "You're too smart to go into primary care."

Since primary care and underserved communities are prominent in the MSM mission, it would be fair to say that the entirety of the curriculum is slanted toward reinforcing students' interest in primary care and nudging them toward underserved communities. Faculty specialists are generally mindful of the school's mission, so the "hidden curriculum" is reduced to a minimum. It is unlikely that top students at MSM have been told that they are too smart to go into primary care.

The MSM curriculum includes a required first-year course in community health that is taught almost entirely in the community for a half day per week throughout the school year (see case study). MSM was one of the first medical schools to assign students to projects in the community (not just to community medical practices). Many schools now have such courses (although they are often electives), and they are becoming more commonplace year by year.

Other features of the curriculum include a first-year Preceptorship Program that sends each student on several half-day visits to community primary care practices and other community health care institutions such as nursing homes and public health centers. Third-year clinical clerkships include outpatient primary care experiences in family medicine, internal medicine, and pediatrics, as well as a rural clerkship. Fourth-year electives include a variety of primary care, rural, and public health opportunities.

A unique honors program in community service extends across the four years of medical school. Students earning an "A" in the first-year community health course are eligible. Those who elect to pursue honors engage in 40 hours of community service in their second year, usually at their Community Health course site. In their third year, they plan a community health promotion project and write a protocol that must be approved by the Honors Committee. In the fourth year, they conduct the project and write and defend (before the committee and others) a thesis that describes and evaluates the project. Students completing the program are noted during commencement exercises to be graduating with honors in community service, and this is recorded on their diplomas.

Location of Clinical Experience

To this modality should be added "and interaction with the community," since a student seeing patients in, for instance, a rural practice may have an experience nearly identical to that of a student seeing patients in a hospital clinic unless he or she interacts with, and learns about, the rural community. This principle is operationalized in the pediatric, family medicine, and rural clerkships through community projects, experiences in community programs such as homeless shelters and soup kitchens, and attending medical society meetings and social programs with faculty preceptors.

Clinical experiences for MSM students include the following:

- Hospital-based clerkships. Third-year required clerkships in internal medicine, obstetrics and gynecology, and surgery are conducted at Grady Memorial Hospital, Atlanta's 896-bed public hospital. The patients there are underserved and beset by

CASE STUDY: The Community Health Course[1]

Since 1998, the Community Health Course has been a requirement for all first-year MSM medical students. Students are assigned to small groups that, over the years, have varied in size from 8 to 16 individuals. Each small group is assigned to a community; the group is based at a school, a church, a Boys and Girls Club, a day care center, or some other community site. The group is supervised by two faculty members—usually a physician and another health professional—and works with a "community liaison," usually an individual who works at the site. The group meets one afternoon per week throughout the school year. During the first semester, the group conducts a community health needs assessment that is driven by the "Clinical Community Health" format,[2] in which the community is considered to be a patient. "Subjective" information is collected through key informant interviews with community leaders, focus groups, and surveys. "Objective" information consists of morbidity, mortality, and demographic data downloaded from health department and census bureau websites, among others, as well as a "windshield survey" (a drive-through or walk-through of the community to observe its features). The students form an assessment, construct a problem list, and develop a plan. The plan is usually a health promotion intervention but may include advocating with public officials for policy change or other activities. At the end of the term, the students, working in teams of two or three, give a presentation (with slides) on the semester's activities.

In the second semester, each group carries out and evaluates a health promotion intervention that addresses one or more of the problems identified in the first semester. The most frequently identified health problems have included violence, substance abuse, and a lack of community development (including unemployment, deteriorating housing, and lack of security). Other frequently identified problems include low literacy rates, obesity and nutritional issues, chronic diseases such as asthma and hypertension, and adolescent sexual health.

References
    1. Buckner, A., Y. D. Ndjakani, B. Banks, and D. S. Blumenthal. 2010. "Using Service-Learning to Teach Community Health: The Morehouse School of Medicine Community Health Course." *Academic Medicine* 85 (10): 1645–51. doi:10.1097 /ACM.0b013e3181f08348.
    2. Blumenthal, D. S. 2009. "Clinical Community Health: Revisiting 'The Community as Patient.'" *Education for Health (Abingdon)* 22 (2): 234.

numerous social as well as medical problems. MSM students, who have heard throughout their first two years of medical education about the social determinants of health, see the effects of social determinants at Grady. It is "traditional" for medical students to learn on the poor so that they can later care for the affluent, but it is also true that if graduates are to care for the underserved, it is best to learn how to do so as students.

- The central element of the required third-year pediatrics clerkship is an ambulatory general pediatrics rotation at the office of a general pediatrician or a federally qualified health center.
- The required family medicine clerkship is housed in the family practice center (officially known as the Comprehensive Family Health Care Center) in East Point, a blue-collar suburb of Atlanta. The patients are nearly all African American.
- The required Rural Health Clerkship, conducted by the Department of Family Medicine, takes place in 15 rural practices and community health centers in medically underserved areas in Georgia. Many of these clerkship experiences are supported by the AHEC Program, described in the "Pipeline" section.
- Student-run clinic. Numerous students voluntarily participate in this clinic each year under faculty supervision. The clinic takes place biweekly in the City of Refuge, a center serving Atlanta's poor and homeless.

Tuition Management

Surveys show that educational debt is a major factor in driving students to high-paying specialties and away from primary care.[34] Financial support is particularly important for MSM students, whose parents' average income is about $66,000 per year, as compared to $117,000 per year among the parents of medical students nationally (2010–15 averages, AAMC data). The average loan debt for MSM medical students is $228,000. About two-thirds of medical students receive scholarships, averaging $8,773 (2018 MSM data).

Mentoring

Strong teacher-student relationships are characteristic of MSM, with both faculty and students remarking in surveys on the "family atmosphere" and "supportive faculty" as key elements of the school's milieu and mentoring. The small class size and low student-faculty ratio were key facilitators of this environment, but as entering class size increased from 24 members of the first class in 1979 to 56 matriculants in 2010, with plans in place to enlarge class size further, concern developed around maintaining this essential feature of the MSM program.

Hence, in 2011 the school launched an initiative entitled "Mentoring Students at Morehouse," or "MSM," the acronym for the school itself. This was a "quality enhancement plan" prepared for the school's reaccreditation by the Southern Association of Colleges and Schools. The goals of the initiative were

1. to assure the success of mentoring programs through ongoing faculty training;
2. to enhance students' academic success by expanding and enriching peer/near-peer mentoring and enhancing the support of challenged students in course enrichment mentoring and tutoring; and
3. to enhance student development as professionals through the establishment of learning communities.

The central component of the plan was the creation of learning communities, small groups of students that meet regularly under the leadership of a seasoned faculty mentor throughout the four years of the medical education program. The groups are the same as the groups in the Community Health course.

An ongoing series of workshops trains faculty in mentoring skills, and learning community leaders are expected to attend. Peer-to-peer mentoring within the learning communities is important as well. Through participation in these communities, students address competencies in teamwork, communication, professionalism, and lifelong learning skills, in addition to being assured of consistent mentoring by faculty.

MSM entering class size has now reached 100 and is projected to remain at that level. Over the years, mentoring and close faculty-student relationships have been given much of the credit for enabling Morehouse students, who enter medical school with lesser academic credentials than those brought by more traditional students, to perform well on national exams and go on to become excellent physicians. Despite the enlarged class size, it seems that mentoring has been able to keep up.

Postgraduate Engagement

The MSM Office of Extended Professional Education offers multiple Accreditation Council on Continuing Medical Education–accredited conferences and programs, as well as literally dozens of nonaccredited online courses. In addition, the AHEC program offers online courses, as well as in-person programs in some of the smaller Georgia cities for the convenience of rural practitioners. But given the number of alternative sources of continuing professional education, a more important resource for physicians practicing in medically underserved areas may be the Georgia Health Information Technology Extension Center (GA-HITEC). This is Georgia's only federally endorsed health information technology center focused on providing technical assistance to providers and hospitals throughout the entire electronic health record (EHR) implementation process and beyond, including assistance with the reporting required to qualify for and receive federal EHR Incentive Program payments. GA-HITEC specializes in working with providers who care for underserved populations in rural and urban areas throughout Georgia. The center has about 4,000 clients.

Social Accountability in Research

Most of the discussion, assessment, and analysis regarding the social accountability of medical schools have been directed at the schools' educational program for medical students. The documents generated by deliberative bodies and organizations refer to "education, research, and service," but the focus is consistently on education and the practice patterns of medical graduates; little attention is given to the social accountability of the schools' research programs (or their service programs, which will be discussed in the next section of this chapter).

The argument that biomedical research programs at medical schools should be socially accountable is much the same as the argument for socially accountable medical education programs: the research programs are primarily supported by public funds, and there is a professional and social ethic that calls on individuals and institutions in medicine to demonstrate altruism and work for the improvement of the health of society. Hence, as stated in the WHO definition cited earlier in this chapter, research should be "directed at the priority health concerns of the community, region, and/or nation that they have a mandate to serve."

If the priority health concerns are those with the highest mortality rates, then the NIH budget adheres roughly to that guideline. For instance, the National Cancer Institute has by far the largest budget of any NIH institute (about $5 billion per year). Institutes dedicated to diseases with very low mortality rates have much smaller budgets. For instance, the budget of the National Eye Institute is about $700 million per year, and that of the National Institute of Arthritis and Musculoskeletal and Skin Diseases is about $550 million per year.

But in the communities with the highest mortality rates, the priority health concerns are likely to be different. There, residents may cite violence, drug abuse, teen pregnancy, or other maladies with social roots as priority health concerns. And even if there is a national consensus that cancer is the most important health problem, the question still remains, what sort of research is most important? Is it molecular research, which may lead to more effective cancer treatments? Or is it community-based prevention research, which may lead to fewer people with cancer?

Moreover, any socially accountable research agenda must include research on racial and ethnic health disparities, and the researchers most likely to address disparities are themselves racial and ethnic minorities. But in 2015, only 6.5 percent of doctorates were earned by African Americans, and only 7.0 percent were awarded to Hispanics.[35]

These issues are addressed at MSM and discussed in chapter 3.

Social Accountability in Service

"Service" at most medical schools refers to clinical service, and most schools view themselves as providers of the most sophisticated specialty care for patients with rare diseases or who are desperately ill. The physician workforce in the United States is heavily tilted toward specialists; as discussed earlier in this chapter, the greatest shortages are in the area of primary care and preventive medicine.

But the most socially accountable health service might not be medical care, but rather health promotion services that can address problems such as obesity, opioid addiction, and HIV infection, which are the causes of much preventable death and disability. There is a focus on this type of service at MSM, and it is described in chapters 4 and 5.

Social Accountability in Public Health

As noted in the brief sections on research and service, most deliberations on social accountability focus on the education and training of future physicians to provide clinical services. Largely omitted from the discussion are public health services, although public health, at least in the traditional sense, is the most socially accountable health service of all. This is because traditional public health is a government service and public health officials are appointed by publicly elected representatives. If the public health system deteriorates, the representatives can be voted out of office.

There are many definitions of public health, but one of the most popular is "what we as a society do collectively to insure the conditions in which people can be healthy."[36] Governmental public health services typically include health-related data collection, health education of the public, screening, immunization, outbreak investigation, and environmental services such as sanitary and restaurant inspections. The services are tax supported and available to everybody, although they often focus on the population groups with the poorest health status.

But not everybody with a public health degree works in traditional governmental public health. The skills learned in earning a public health degree can be applied in managing a large medical practice or other health services organization, in analyzing data for an insurance company, in conducting research for a pharmaceutical company, or in numerous other capacities that are not part of what we usually consider public health.

Master's and doctoral degree programs in public health are by the nature of public health socially accountable, but some are more so than others. Large schools of public health may have hundreds of master of public health (MPH) students and dozens of doctoral students. This large size does not necessarily obviate social accountability—large programs may still prepare their graduates to address the priority health problems of a community, region, or nation—but it creates a challenge. Medical schools or other colleges and universities may also offer MPH programs, and these are typically smaller than those housed in schools of public health. The MSM MPH program, with about 60 students, is one of these.

The social accountability of an MPH program (or a doctor of public health program) could be evaluated using the same "Beyond Flexner" modalities as described earlier in this chapter for doctor of medicine (MD) programs. The following briefly describes MSM's MPH program.

Mission

The MSM MPH program shares the school's mission, and this is cited often by faculty and referenced frequently in the program's written and online materials. MSM offers not only MD and MPH degrees but several master's degree programs and a PhD program in the basic sciences. Hence, the MSM mission statement, rather than focusing on the education of physicians, states that the school will "increase the diversity of the health professional and scientific workforce" and refers to primary *health* care rather than primary medical care. However, the MPH program does have its own mission statement: to develop, through graduate education, public health leaders who are fluent in community-focused public health practice, particularly in underserved communities.

Pipeline

The MPH program relies on and benefits from the same pipeline as the medical education program. As described earlier, pipeline programs promote STEAM rather than medicine, and the AHEC program is relentlessly interdisciplinary.

Admissions

The challenge in MPH admissions is screening out those applicants who have no real interest in public health but think that an MPH degree will strengthen their credentials for medical school admission. (However, MPH graduates who go on to medical school will likely become physicians with a greater appreciation of, and orientation to, public health.) Just as the MSM MD Admissions Committee takes applicants' college grades and MCAT scores into consideration but then searches for essential "noncognitive" qualities, so the MSM MPH Admissions Committee takes applicants' college grades and scores on the Graduate Record Exam into consideration but then searches for characteristics that fit the MPH program's emphasis on community-focused public health and concern for health equity.

It should be noted that 80–90 percent of MSM MPH students are African American, and almost all of the remainder are Hispanic or another minority. The program views its most significant diversity challenge as recruiting more males. The percentage of male students hovers around 40 percent but has sunk as low as 14 percent in one class. This reflects the gender disparity in higher education generally, but the disparity is even greater among African Americans than among the population at large.

Curriculum

All accredited MPH programs are required to have core courses in epidemiology, biostatistics, behavioral health, environmental health, and health administration and policy. Beyond the core, individual programs have much flexibility and discretion. The MSM MPH program is distinguished by courses that reflect its mission and its substantial practicum requirement.

Location of Practicum (Replacing "Clinical Experience" in the Beyond Flexner Modalities)

MPH accreditation requirements promulgated by the Council on Education for Public Health specify an "Applied Practice Experience," or APE, for each MPH student.[37] Very broad latitude is allowed regarding the setting of the experience and its length. The MSM MPH program, because of its community focus, requires that the practicum experience be in the community (at a community agency or organization) and that the experience be at least 480 hours in duration (the equivalent of 40 hours per week for 12 weeks, although the experience need not necessarily be done in a solid 12-week block). The APE is composed of two components:

1. Fieldwork: 120-hour blocks at multiple sites or 360 hours at a single site
2. Community service: 120 hours of engagement with MSM MPH

Tuition Management

MSM has managed to keep graduate study tuition rates quite low compared to other private schools. However, as noted in the section on the MD education program at MSM, the parents of Morehouse students generally lack the resources of parents of students attending private schools of public health. Scholarships are thus important, and the program has increased its pool of scholarship funds each year.

Mentoring

The small size of the MSM MPH program helps foster a family atmosphere, and this sense of an MPH family is a particularly salient feature of the program. Advisors are assigned, but small class sizes also facilitate the ability of students to identify mentors themselves. In addition, the program offers specialized learning communities, similar to those in the MD education program: discussion groups of students led by faculty mentors and focusing on topics of student interest, such as time management, self-awareness, study skills, professional development, work/life balance, and motivation. In addition to the student learning communities, there are learning communities for recent graduates, older students, parents, and men.

Postgraduate Engagement

The MSM National Alumni Association includes all MSM alumni—MD, MPH, PhD, and MS. This is rather unique among American institutions of higher education; the norm is for the medical school, the school of public health, the other professional programs, and the undergraduate college each to have its own alumni association. The MSM arrangement reflects the solidarity among MSM students and the "family atmosphere" of the school: academic ceremonies, social events, fundraisers, and so on include all the students, and those that include faculty include the entire faculty.

Social Accountability in International Work

MSM has only a very small international footprint compared to a number of other medical schools and schools of public health that have extensive programs of teaching and research in developing countries. In all of its international programs, however, the school attempts to adhere to the principles that have guided its domestic programs of community engagement. For instance, MSM is a partner of PROMETRA (Promocion de la Medicina Tradicional Amazonica), an international nongovernmental organization headquartered in Dakar, Senegal, whose purpose is to preserve African traditional medicine.[38] An MSM team worked with faculty at Stellenbosch University (Cape Town, South Africa) to develop and evaluate the first AHEC program outside of the

United States. MSM faculty teach in Ghana, and students take advantage of for-credit and noncredit elective opportunities in Haiti, Ghana, and elsewhere.[39]

Summary

The social accountability (or social mission) movement is relatively new, and only in the twenty-first century has it begun to gain traction. The United States seems to lag most of the world in paying it heed. But in view of the support given to medical schools by US society—both financial and through an implicit social contract—the United States should be a leader. However, it is particularly in the United States that students are driven away from the elements of social accountability by the cost of medical education and by the hidden curriculum, both of which influence their career choices.

Several sets of criteria have been developed for evaluating the extent to which a medical school is socially accountable. These are generally process measures, often quite detailed, that focus on those elements of a school's educational program that are thought to lead to socially accountable outcomes. In the end, it is those outcomes that are most important, and they can be summarized as follows:

- Do a high percentage of graduates enter specialties that are most needed? In the United States, those are the primary care specialties.
- Do a high percentage of graduates practice in those communities where they are most needed? In the United States (and elsewhere), these are underserved rural communities and low-income urban communities, often populated by racial and ethnic minorities.
- Are a high percentage of graduate members of population groups underrepresented in medicine? These are the physicians most likely to practice in underserved communities and most likely to be culturally competent with respect to members of their own ethnicity.

- Do the school's research programs focus on the priority health problems of the communities to which they are accountable, and do they partner with those communities in identifying and addressing the priority health problems?
- Do the school's service programs in the areas of medical care and health promotion serve the needs of the communities to which they are accountable, and do they partner with those communities in identifying the needs and governing the services?

The affirmative answers to these questions characterize MSM and are the factors that have led to its recognition as a socially accountable medical school.

References

1. Dictionary.com, s.v. "accountable." http://www.dictionary.com/browse /accountable?s=t.

2. Roskoski, R., Jr. "Ranking Tables of NIH Funding to US Medical Schools in 2017." Blue Ridge Institute for Medical Research. http://www.brimr.org/NIH _Awards/2017/NIH_Awards_2017.htm.

3. Hirsch, Jules. 1969. "Social Responsibility of Medical Schools." *Archives of Internal Medicine* 124 (1): 113–14. doi:10.1001/archinte.1969.00300170115022.

4. Boelen, Charles, and Jeffery E. Heck. 1995. *Defining and Measuring the Social Accountability of Medical Schools.* Geneva: World Health Organization.

5. Health Canada Steering Committee on Social Accountability of Medical Schools. 2001. *Social Accountability: A Vision for Canadian Medical Schools.* Ottawa: Health Canada.

6. Ritz, Stacey, Kathleen Beatty, and Rachel Ellaway. 2014. "Accounting for Social Accountability: Developing Critiques of Social Accountability within Medical Education." *Education for Health* 27 (2): 152–57. doi:10.4103/1357-6283.143747.

7. Buchman, Sandy, Robert Woollard, Ryan Meili, and Ritika Goel. 2016. "Practising Social Accountability: From Theory to Action." *Canadian Family Physician Medecin de famille canadien* 62 (1): 15–18.

8. "Committee on Accreditation of Canadian Medical Schools." https://cacms -cafmc.ca/.

9. Strasser, R., J. C. Hogenbirk, B. Minore, D. C. Marsh, S. Berry, W. G. Mcready, and L. Graves. 2013. "Transforming Health Professional Education through Social Accountability: Canada's Northern Ontario School of Medicine." *MedTeach* 35 (6): 490–96.

10. Campbell, Catherine, Susan A. Papp, and Aparajita Gogoi. 2013. "Improving Maternal Health through Social Accountability: A Case Study from Orissa, India." *Global Public Health* 8 (4): 449–64. doi:10.1080/17441692.2012.748085.

11. Mahoney, Sarah, Linnea Boileau, John Floridis, Christina Abi-Abdallah, and Bernard Lee. 2014. "How Social Accountability Can Be Incorporated into an Urban

Community-Based Medical Education Program: An Australian Initiative." *Education for Health* 27 (2): 148–51. doi:10.4103/1357-6283.143746.

12. Galukande, Moses, Noeline Nakasujja, and Nelson K. Sewankambo. 2012. "Social Accountability: A Survey of Perceptions and Evidence of Its Expression at a Sub Saharan African University." *BMC Medical Education* 12:96. doi:10.1186/1472-6920-12-96.

13. McCrea, Marie Louise, and Deborah Murdoch-Eaton. 2014. "How Do Undergraduate Medical Students Perceive Social Accountability?" *Medical Teacher* 36 (10): 867–75. doi:10.3109/0142159X.2014.916784.

14. Kaufman, A. 2016. "Beyond Flexner Alliance: Social Mission in Health Professions Education." *Education for Health* 29 (3): 277–78.

15. Petterson, Stephen M., Winston R. Liaw, Robert L. Phillips Jr., David L. Rabin, David S. Meyers, and Andrew W. Bazemore. 2012. "Projecting US Primary Care Physician Workforce Needs: 2010–2025." *Annals of Family Medicine* 10 (6): 503–9. doi:10.1370/afm.1431.

16. Abayasekara, Allison. 2015. "Addressing Clinician Workforce Shortages in Underserved Areas." *Journal of Health Care for the Poor and Underserved* 26 (1): 1–4.

17. Committee on Training Physicians for Public Health Careers, Board on Population Health and Public Health Practice, Institute of Medicine, National Academy of Sciences. 2007. *Training Physicians for Public Health Careers.* Washington, DC: National Academies Press.

18. Centers for Disease Control and Prevention. 2013. "CDC Health Disparities and Inequalities Report." In *Morbidity and Mortality Weekly Report.* https://www.cdc.gov/mmwr/preview/mmwrhtml/su6203a2.htm.

19. Komaromy, Miriam, Kevin Grumbach, Michael Drake, Karen Vranizan, Nicole Lurie, Dennis Keane, and Andrew B. Bindman. 1996. "The Role of Black and Hispanic Physicians in Providing Health Care for Underserved Populations." *New England Journal of Medicine* 334:1305–10. doi:10.1056/NEJM199605163342006.

20. US Department of Health and Human Services. 1985. *Report of the Secretary's Task Force on Black and Minority Health.* Washington, DC: US Government Printing Office. O-174-719.

21. "Global Consensus for Social Accountability of Medical Schools." http://healthsocialaccountability.org/.

22. "The Training for Health Equity Network." www.thenetcommunity.org.

23. Ross, Simone, Robyn Preston, Iris Lindemann, Marie Matte, Rex Samson, Filedito Tandinco, Sarah Larkins, Bjorg Palsdottir, and Andre-Jacques Neusy. 2014. "The Training for Health Equity Network Evaluation Framework: A Pilot Study at Five Health Professional Schools." *Education for Health* 27 (2): 116–26. doi:10.4103/1357-6283.143727.

24. Larkins, Sarah L., Robyn Preston, Marie C. Matte, Iris C. Lindemann, Rex Samson, Filedito D. Tandinco, David Buso, Simone J. Ross, Björg Pálsdóttir, and André-Jacques Neusy, on behalf of the Training for Health Equity Network. 2013. "Measuring Social Accountability in Health Professional Education: Development and International Pilot Testing of an Evaluation Framework." *Medical Teacher* 35 (1): 32–45. doi:10.3109/0142159X.2012.731106.

25. Rourke, James. 2018. "Social Accountability: A Framework for Medical Schools to Improve the Health of the Populations They Serve." *Academic Medicine* 93 (8): 1120–24. doi:10.1097/acm.0000000000002239.

26. "ASPIRE Recognition of Excellence in Social Accountability of a Medical School." https://aspire-to-excellence.org/downloads/1348/ASPIRE_REVISED_SA _CRITERIA_2018_Final.pdf.

27. Mullan, Fitzhugh, Candice Chen, Stephen Petterson, Gretchen Kolsky, and Michael Spagnola. 2010. "The Social Mission of Medical Education: Ranking the Schools." *Annals of Internal Medicine* 152 (12): 804–11. doi:10.7326/0003-4819-152-12-201006150-00009.

28. See http://beyondflexner.org/wp-content/uploads/2015/04/Beyond-Flexner -MSM-Final-Report1.pdf.

29. See https://socialmissionmetrics.gwhwi.org.

30. Morley, C. P., E. M. Mader, T. Smilnak, Bazemore, S. Petterson, J. E. Rodríguez, and K. M. Campbell. 2015. "The Social Mission in Medical School Mission Statements: Associations with Graduate Outcomes." *Family Medicine* 47 (6): 427–34.

31. MacDowell, Martin, Michael Glasser, and Matthew Hunsaker. 2013. "A Decade of Rural Physician Workforce Outcomes for the Rockford Rural Medical Education (RMED) Program, University of Illinois." *Academy of Medicine* 88 (12): 1941–47.

32. MacQueen, Ian T., Melinda Maggard-Gibbons, Gina Capra, Laura Raaen, Jesus G. Ulloa, Paul G. Shekelle, Isomi Miake-Lye, Jessica M. Beroes, and Susanne Hempel. 2018. "Recruiting Rural Healthcare Providers Today: A Systematic Review of Training Program Success and Determinants of Geographic Choices." *Journal of General Internal Medicine* 33 (2): 191–99. doi:10.1007/s11606-017-4210-z.

33. Martimianakis, Maria A., Barret Michalec, Justin Lam, Carrie Cartmill, Janelle S. Taylor, and Frederic W. Hafferty. 2015. "Humanism, the Hidden Curriculum, and Educational Reform: A Scoping Review and Thematic Analysis." *Academy of Medicine* 90 (S11): S5–13.

34. Phillips, Julie. 2013. *Educational Debt and Career Choice: Every Student Matters.* Vol. 45.

35. National Science Foundation, National Center for Science and Engineering Statistics Directorate for Social, Behavioral and Economic Sciences. 2015. *2015 Doctorate Recipients from U.S. Universities.*

36. Institute of Medicine. 1988. *The Future of Public Health.* Washington, DC: National Academies Press.

37. Council on Education for Public Health. 2016. *Accreditation Criteria: Schools of Public Health and Public Health Programs.* Silver Spring, MD: Council on Education for Public Health. https://ceph.org/assets/2016.Criteria.pdf.

38. See https://prometra.org/.

39. Moodley, K., T. H. Akintobi, T. Fish, and D. S. Blumenthal. 2018. "A Pipeline Program to Address the South African Crisis in Human Resources for Health." *Annals of Global Health* 84:66–76. doi:http://doi.org/10.29024/aogh.12.

THREE

Community-Based Participatory Research

D ESPITE NOTEWORTHY advances in the health status of the US population, racial/ethnic minority and other health disparity populations experience a higher proportion of chronic and infectious diseases compared to other groups.[1,2] The United States is at a critical juncture in advancing health equity through research, as well as policy, systems, and environmental change strategies designed to reduce health disparities.[3] Identifying effective multilevel strategies requires local understanding of community or neighborhood context in order to develop approaches that are community led, implemented, and sustained. What follows is a description of community engagement research systematically built and scaled over time and based on community-based participatory research (CBPR) principles adapted in local contexts.

Community-Based Participatory Research: An Art, Science, and Practice

CBPR emphasizes the fostering, deployment, and sustaining of community-academic partnerships that share leadership in the planning, implementation, evaluation, and dissemination of "innovative, culturally appropriate and evidence-based interventions that enhance translation of research findings for community and policy change."[4, 5] It is distinct in that it involves the intentional elevation of community or patient stakeholder groups, among others, capitalizing on their unique strengths and perspectives. Community may be defined in myriad ways that include, but are not limited, to a common geography, identity, or lived experience, whether innate, chosen, or otherwise experienced. Together partners address mutually identified priorities and research questions in response. Outcomes include both statistically significant research results and practically significant responses to the more immediate social services and needs or the politically rooted systems that created health disparities and inequities. A CBPR approach has been advocated and promulgated at Morehouse School of Medicine (MSM) and has been closely interdigitated with the Morehouse Model for CE.

Among the advantages of CBPR are neighborhood-campus trust and relationships; improved relevance of research questions; enhanced research recruitment; contextually relevant (and more effective) interventions; increased collaborative research capacities among communities, academic institutions, and agencies; and changes in the traditionally and historically unequal power dynamics among diverse stakeholder groups.[6–11] A tenet of CBPR is that researchers who want to conduct effective public health research must invest time and resources in building partnerships with community-based organizations and/or neighborhood residents who are gatekeepers to establishing and maintaining community buy-in, ownership, and sustainability. Ideally, community residents are equal or senior partners throughout the research process.[12]

While the benefits of CBPR have been well documented,[8, 13–16] there are challenges in building and maintaining research partnerships between community and academic researchers. Academic researchers, who have been traditionally trained to conduct "independent" or "investigator-initiated" research, often make unilateral decisions and consequently have poor participatory communication skills (e.g., making decisions without input or infrequent communication). There are also few incentives for community engagement in academia, and historically community-engaged research efforts have not been duly recognized as part of the tenure and promotion reward systems in the academy. As a result, limited time is typically spent developing and committing to the partnership, even among those who may want to establish such research partnerships.[16, 17] As a result, even when research is carried out in community settings, there may be little if any input from or engagement of community residents, beyond requests to participate in a study or clinical trial. Plans for sustaining the intervention are unsuccessful because information flow back to communities is less of a priority, as is the translation of this knowledge to lay audiences.[18–20] Community residents and leaders have less familiarity with research, processes, and requirements related to the institutional review boards and research designs. Moreover, research mistrust due to personal negative experiences and/or the national and global residue associated with the historical mistreatment of minority populations by researchers (e.g., the Tuskegee Syphilis Study, the Nuremburg Trials, Henrietta Lacks) are understandably still pervasive.[21–23]

The MSM Prevention Research Center Community Coalition Board

Establishing a governing body that ensures community-based participation in research is challenging when (1) academicians have not previously been guided by neighborhood leaders in understanding a community's ecology, (2) community members have not led discussions regarding their health priorities, or (3) academics and neighborhood leaders have not historically worked together as a single body with established rules to guide roles and operations.[8, 12, 24–26] Further, communities that may have experienced exploitation in research or other social systems (economic, political, racial/ethnic) all the more deserve a place at the research development and implementation table toward actionable responses that they co-create.

The MSM Prevention Research Center (PRC), funded by the Centers for Disease Control and Prevention in 1998, strongly holds to the applied definition of CBPR, in that it is dynamic, is "tailor-made," focuses on prevention, establishes partnerships between communities and research entities, develops improved interventions that are culturally focused, and establishes effective health policies addressing health disparities and inequities. This definition has been applied to myriad clinical, social, behavioral, and translational research, as well as other collaborative public health training, practice, and evaluation initiatives since the PRC's founding.[27–47] National recognition for the PRC's leadership in community-engaged applied public health and prevention has included the first Annual Award from Community-Campus Partnerships for Health (2002), the CDC's Outstanding Community-Based Participatory Research Award (2004) and the CDC's Excellence in Community-Based Research Award for the MSM PRC's Community Coalition Board (CCB; 2005), the Georgia Healthcare Foundation 2010 Joseph D. Greene Community Service Award for continued extraordinary commitment to improving the quality of health and health care, and the 2017 Lucille Webb Award in recognition for dedication and commitment to building and sustaining community-engaged partnerships. The PRC's mission is to advance scientific knowledge in the field of prevention in African American and other minority communities and to disseminate new information and strategies for prevention.

The PRC's integrated research and translation agenda capitalizes on community wisdom and that of translation partners to attend to the multilevel influences on health outcomes that result in health inequities. These inequities are unnecessary, avoidable, unfair, and unjust and are rooted in social injustices (including policies, systems and environments) that make some population groups more vulnerable to poor health than others.[1] In order to effectively scale up and adapt MSM PRC scientific discoveries into public health practice and advance health equity, we strategically translate evidence-based research for diverse minority and health disparity populations.[2]

In our guiding framework, minority and other health disparity communities experiencing the burden of health inequity are positioned as senior partners in planning, developing, and evaluating research, center intervention strategies, and implementation using the PRC's CCB research leadership model, which will be described later.

The CBPR mind-set of MSM PRC founders necessitated the identification of strategic alliances capitalizing on existing community strengths found in neighborhood planning units (NPUs).[2, 48–51] The city of Atlanta is divided into 25 NPUs within which citizen advisory councils are organized. These citizen advisory councils make recommendations to the mayor and city council on zoning, land use, and other planning issues. The NPU governance structure represented a preexisting neighborhood leadership infrastructure for CBPR relationship development from the inception of the PRC.[25] Five contiguous NPUs in southwest Atlanta are PRC partners.

The demographic characteristics of the PRC research partner communities (RPCs) help explain their increased incidence and prevalence of both chronic and infectious disease. At the aggregate level, 88 percent of the residents are young African Americans (median age = 30 years) with low educational attainment (26% of adults have not completed high school), and they are ranked among the lowest with respect to a constellation of neighborhood health and quality of life indicators among the 25 NPUs.[52, 53] Major causes of morbidity are cardiovascular diseases, respiratory diseases, mental and behavioral disorders, and human immunodeficiency virus (HIV)/AIDS.[54]

Atlanta community members of the CCB initially expressed their apprehension about participating in yet another partnership with an academic institution to conduct what they perceived as meaningless research in their neighborhoods. In order to flip this script toward community leadership in research, at the outset the PRC created a governance model in which the community would serve as the "senior partner" in its relationship with the medical school and other academic and agency collaborators. The CCB was structured as a *policy-making* board for the PRC rather than as an "advisory board." In efforts to reduce health inequities in underserved communities, the PRC has strategically partnered with the CCB and partner communities to conduct health research and carry out interventions designed with or led by community leaders.

Even the location of the PRC had both symbolic meaning and practical implications resulting from one of its earliest policies. Locating the PRC in the community served is a *requirement* of the PRC's CCB. This provides daily interaction with CCB members and community access to center resources, such as meeting space, supplies, and technology. The PRC is located in office space in one of its partner communities five miles south of the medical school campus. These resources democratize access and facilitate engagement between neighborhood residents and academic faculty and staff was perceived to be more limited if the PRC were located behind the main campus's gates.

The CCB has served as the *governing body* for the PRC since 1999. The board is composed of 23 members representing three member types: neighborhood residents (16 seats; always in majority number), academic institutions (3 seats), and health/social service agencies (4 seats). The board has met bimonthly (every two months) since inception. Community representatives hold the preponderance of power, literally putting them at the forefront of all CBPR and related approaches. Board members, including academic, agency, and neighborhood representatives, truly represent the community and its priorities. Academic representatives are faculty frequently engaged in carrying out the research, service, or training initiatives affiliated with the PRC. Each type of agency was strategically selected owing to its significance in addressing the social determinants of health, including, but not limited to, local health services, education, and affordable housing.[3]

The CCB bylaws stipulate, in addition to the required neighborhood representative majority on the board, that the board chair, vice chair, and secretary must always be neighborhood representatives. Hence, in any vote that pits the neighborhoods against the academics and public health professionals, the neighborhoods would have the most votes (however, this has never occurred). The neighborhoods represented are identified through the NPUs. Corresponding community values, research priorities, and evaluation criteria were created shortly after the PRC was established and have been ratified over time (see table 3.1).[55, 56]

The role of the CCB is to (*a*) set policy and oversee the operations of the PRC, (*b*) identify priorities and approve projects, (*c*) provide information on center activities to the organizations and agencies represented on the board, and (*d*) develop a strategic plan to guide the PRC's long-term objectives. The CCB holds center faculty and staff accountable by setting policies and priorities; approving, actively engaging in, and

Table 3.1 MSM PRC Community Values, Research Priorities, and Evaluation Criteria

Community Values Reflecting the Cultural Context of Approved Research Projects

1. Policies and programs should be based on mutual respect and justice for all people, free from discrimination or bias.

2. All people have a right to political, economic, cultural, and environmental self-determination.

3. The community has the right to participate as an equal partner at every level of decision-making, including needs assessment, planning, implementation, enforcement, and evaluation.

4. Principles of individual and community-informed consent should be strictly enforced.

5. The community repudiates the targeting of people of color and lower socioeconomic status in research of all types without full knowledge of their rights and consent.

6. Present and future generations should be provided an education that emphasizes social and environmental issues, based on our experience and an appreciation of our diverse cultural perspectives.

7. Research processes and outcomes should benefit the community. Community members should be hired and trained whenever possible and appropriate, and the research should help build and enhance community assets.

8. Community members should participate in all aspects of research from conceptualization to dissemination of findings.

9. Productive partnerships between researchers and community members should be encouraged to last beyond the life of the project. This will make it more likely that research findings will be incorporated into ongoing community programs and therefore provide the greatest possible benefit to the community from research.

10. Community members should be empowered to initiate their own research projects, which address needs they identify themselves.

Research Priorities

1. Projects that, if successful, will contribute to a reduction in the disparity in health status between the White population and the African American or other minority population.

2. Projects that, if successful, will contribute to improving the health status of African American males.

3. Projects that, if successful, will reduce injustice, including environmental injustice.

Evaluation Criteria

1. Projects should not violate community values or standards.

2. They should have the potential to benefit the community through a health promotion intervention. Projects that propose simply to gather data should include in the proposal information on how the data-gathering process will lead to an intervention or otherwise improve the health of the community.

3. Their effectiveness should be subject to evaluation and, if effectiveness can be demonstrated, they should be replicable in another setting.

monitoring research; and actively leading or partnering in evaluation, communication, and dissemination. The CCB integration in directing the PRC's work is detailed in table 3.2.

In the context of CBPR, a CCB, composed of local stakeholders who serve and reside in prioritized communities, adds substance to research and other health initiatives by providing local leadership and guidance on the most appropriate positioning of interventions, modes of community engagement for data collection, and access to neighborhood residents and leaders critical to effective public health initiatives.[12] Ideally, community residents should be equal or senior partners in relation to academic stakeholders on such boards, informing the development of the evaluation question, the logic model, appropriate recruitment and retention strategies, and, most importantly, the translation of results to inform decision-making, policy change, or subsequent research.[57]

Table 3.2 Community Coalition Board Level of Involvement in MSM PRC Center and Research

Key element	CCB level of involvement
Research	Establishes core research agenda; establishes research priorities; reviews all projects and protocols; may modify or reject a project/protocol; community-engaged research committees (deployed to lead specific research projects from conception to dissemination); leads community-engaged research
Communication	Serves as subject matter expert on topic development for presentations, workshops, webinars, media, and web/social media content and/or messaging; coauthors manuscripts and written documents, e.g., journal articles, bulletins, fact sheets; presents findings and promotes health at scientific and community presentations, on radio, on TV, and through other media and social media outlets; disseminates research findings and health materials in communities served by PRC; and serves on Communications and Technology Committee (established in 2010 and co-chaired by CCB member); 20 newsletters; 80 radio shows
Training	Supports recruitment of CHW personnel; co-leads students and community courses and trainings on designated PRC research priority topics established by the CCB
Evaluation	Co-leads development of surveys for appropriate data collection; participating in and leading data collection; presenting evaluation findings in community and academic setting; providing input as CCB member in the PRC's collection of data from the CCB; and assisting in programmatic decision-making based on evaluation findings that impact the PRC and/or the CCB; and serving on the Data Monitoring and Evaluation Committee (established in 2011 and co-chaired by CCB member)

Prior to the development and maintenance of such a board, it is important to distinguish between community *advisory* and *governance* boards. The primary similarity between these boards is that representatives may be narrowly or broadly selected based on the needs of the research or health initiative. Advisory board members work together for research teams designed to garner community representation "in the development of a research agenda and research processes . . . to advise on study design and implementation, facilitate community consent, evaluate and communicate the risks and benefits of research, evaluate education materials and disseminate information."[58, 59] Members serving in an *advisory role* "provide information, guidance, or suggestions from the community that the research team may choose to accept or reject." The PRC CCB model detailed earlier provides a specific example of a community research *governance* model, complete with *collectively* (community, academic, and agency member) developed bylaws, research priorities, and evaluation criteria. More generally, community members of governance or coalition boards function in the role of *partners with* rather than advisors to researchers. They bring issues and concerns to and from the community toward mutually beneficial resolutions or strategies based on a relationship that has been built and established over time. The relationship is, ideally, not based on a single funded initiative.

Central to *establishing* such a board was an iterative process of disagreement, dialogue, and compromise that ultimately resulted in the identification of what academicians needed from neighborhood board members and what the academics, in turn, would offer communities. Not unlike other new social exchanges, each partner had to first learn, respect, and then value what the other considered a worthy benefit in return for participating on the board.[57, 60] According to a former PRC CCB chair, community members allowed researchers conditional access to their communities to engage in research that had an established community benefit. Benefits to CCB members, in addition to the research findings, include building of research and evaluation skills and an increased ability to access and navigate clinical and social services.[28–30] Among benefits to academic researchers are (1) established community trust and (2) relationships with partners who have direct connections to local strengths (leaders and resources) central to advancing health equity.

Critical to *maintaining* a community-driven governing board are bylaws that provide a blueprint for the governing body. Board members should be people who truly represent the community and its priorities whenever possible. The differing values of academic and community CCB representatives are acknowledged and coexist within an established infrastructure that supports collective functioning to address community health promotion initiatives.[12, 61] Lessons learned in CBPR CCB development and sustainability are detailed below:

- Engagement in effective CCBs is developed through multidirectional learning of each partner's values and needs.[26]
- CCBs are built and sustained over time to ensure community ownership through established rules and governance structures.
- Trust and relationship building are both central to the ability of neighborhood and research experts to work together to shape community-engaged research agendas.
- Maintaining a CCB requires ongoing communication and feedback, beyond formal monthly or quarterly meetings, to keep members engaged.
- Both fiscal and nonfiscal acknowledgment of community members as *partners* (beyond the roles of research participants) should be institutionalized at the beginning of the partnership given historical and current imbalances in academic and community power.

The CCB research leadership model has been adapted to other local and statewide networks of academic researchers working in collaboration with community residents through the Centers of Excellence on Health Disparities (funded by the National Institutes of Health [NIH] from 2011 to 2016), the Atlanta Clinical and Translational Science Institute (funded by NIH from 2007 to 2017), and its successor, the Georgia Clinical and Translational Science Alliance (Georgia CTSA; funded by NIH from 2017 to 2022), as described in the following sections.

CBPR-Driven Community Health Needs Assessments to Catalyze Action

The PRC has strategically partnered with the communities to facilitate health research and related interventions informed in large part by community health needs assessments (CHNAs) conducted every four years by CCB members and center staff. These assessments differ from those conducted in "usual practice," which are characterized by disease statistics, with little or no attention to social determinants of health. Social determinants of health are now recognized as central to understanding and developing interventions that address root causes and advance health equity.[3, 62] Although more recently reported CHNAs have infused community voices, few have reported how results have advanced related research or responsive interventions.[63–66] The PRC CHNA process is designed to (1) collect and analyze qualitative and quantitative data from community stakeholders and secondary data sources to identify health needs, priorities, and perceptions to inform research and intervention implementation and (2) use recommendations for planning and implementing research projects, disease prevention activities, health promotion outreach, and evaluation initiatives in support of a CBPR agenda.

Following MSM Institutional Review Board (IRB) approval, all CHNA activities, from survey development to data analyses, are reviewed, monitored, and evaluated by the CCB at large and by its Data Monitoring and Evaluation Committee (DMEC). The DMEC, established in 2011, was designed to extend CBPR engagement of CCB members in the work of the PRC. The DMEC (eight members) has academic-community co-leadership (a CCB neighborhood resident member and the MSM PRC assistant director for evaluation) and is tasked with leading the assessment functions of the PRC. Members meet bimonthly (every other month, during months when the CCB does not meet) to discuss and inform CHNA evaluation activities, inform data collection planning and implementation, and prepare for reporting of evaluation findings and interim results to the broader CCB, where data collection processes and challenges are presented and recommendations are sought and acted on.

CHNA Primary Data Collection Tool Development

The PRC and CCB (led by the DMEC) implement a systematic approach to update the previously administered CHNA. RPC focus groups are conducted to review survey length and ensure culturally relevant and resonant wording, comprehension, and face validity. CCB members participate in a one-hour training conducted by PRC staff to ensure consistent survey administration. CCB members receive $25.00 for attending data collection training and up to $25.00 for the return of completed surveys to the PRC for analysis. This is in addition to ongoing fiscal acknowledgment of time for each CCB community member's participation in each two-hour bimonthly meeting. The CCB identifies other community leaders with networks who are also invited to participate in training toward leadership in survey administration. They receive the same fiscal acknowledgment of time for completion of training and submission of completed surveys.

The concept of fiscal renumeration for community members' engagement as partners in research development and implementation (beyond roles as research participants) is still evolving in the literature.[67] CBPR benefits and challenges are well detailed in the literature, but there is a newer and limited blueprint on how this equity translates into models for community incentives, "payment," or compensation beyond the fundamental paths toward and outcomes of building and maintaining trust and respect and sharing power, benefits, and leadership.[68-71] The well-acknowledged imbalance of power between academic and health disparity community partners is steeped in institutionalized inequalities based on race and socioeconomic status, among many other factors. These are among the inequities that CBPR approaches are designed to address. It is this imbalance and appreciation that necessitated establishment of fiscal acknowledgment for CCB members and other community partners since 2010. This was made possible by an institutional endowment and prioritization of the CBPR leadership of the PRC. In the context of the PRC, we positioned incentives as a *basic* acknowledgment, rather than payment, for CCB member engagement. Community partners' time, talents, and expertise are priceless. This fiscal acknowledgment is still unequal and not righted by this renumeration. Well-intended CBPR-based partners still grapple with how to navigate the institutionalized red tape that can make payments to any nonacademic partner difficult.

A two-pronged survey administration process from a convenience sample of residents is implemented following biostatistician consultation to ensure representative community sample size targets. While a convenience sample traditionally limits generalizability, this sampling strategy is justified for implementation of a locally relevant CHNA process to facilitate and inform CBPR through the trust to build and sustain community engagement. The intention to strategically engage community residents who would not otherwise engage in research necessitates the use of a convenience sample. Both the CCB and community leaders lead this process, as trusted gatekeepers and CBOs that have established relationships (nonresearch) with residents. First, CCB members and research center staff administer surveys at neighborhood meetings, recreational facilities, senior centers, and health clinics. Residents who complete surveys face-to-face through this approach receive nonmonetary incentives (i.e., pedometers or tote bags) for their participation. Second, the MSM uses email and social media platforms to allow residents to anonymously complete surveys. Email messages with an electronic survey link are also sent to neighborhood listservs.

Center staff mine secondary data from multiple sources, including state and local health departments (e.g., Georgia Department of Public Health Online Analytical Statistical Information System database), community-serving organizations (e.g., City of Atlanta Department of Planning and Community Development), and partner agencies and institutions (e.g., Atlanta Housing Authority). The secondary data inform development of a community profile. Review of these sources is central to comparison of community perceptions and experiences to local health status indices.

Community Engagement in Data Analysis and Interpretation Guiding Core Research

The DMEC reviews, prepares, and presents CHNA results to the full CCB body at its annual retreat. This forum is selected because members annually spend a day together to reflect and interpret center data, processes, systems, and outcomes to set the PRC's direction. In response to CHNA data indicating that Black youth in Georgia bear a disproportionate burden of sexually transmitted infections (STIs) and HIV infection, a research study, entitled *A Multi-method Approach to STI and HIV/AIDS Prevention among Urban Minority Youth*, was conceived and subsequently implemented (2014–19). The study features its own youth community leadership board, explores the effectiveness of a multicomponent intervention on STI and HIV/AIDS prevention efforts among teens, and builds on prior research reviewed and prioritized by the CCB.

Community Action Planning by Project Review Committee

PRC faculty, staff, and CCB agree that CHNA alignment would be among the initial determinants of any proposed health initiative or project. If a proposed research project or health initiative meets this criterion, the CCB chair assigns a project review committee. This committee, composed of two or three CCB members with content expertise or interest, discusses the research or health initiative concept and alignment with the board's community values and has the authority to require modification of the project or even to disapprove it. The project review committee model has been strategically employed over time to (1) systematically review and prioritize interventions; (2) advance policy, systems, and environmental change approaches through community-clinical linkages; and (3) fund community-led grants and job creation. Table 3.3 details the outcomes of the CBPR-driven CHNA. Cardiovascular disease and diabetes concerns were addressed through a policy, systems, and environmental approach addressing the risks, including limited access to opportunities for safe physical activity and access to low-cost healthy food.[31, 46, 72]

Table 3.3 PRC Community Health Needs Assessment—Health Concerns, Causes, Solutions, and Response

Issue/concern	Causes	Solutions	PRC response
Cardiovascular disease (CVD)/ hypertension/high blood pressure	"eating habits" "lack of knowledge" "salty/fatty foods" "stress" "too much sodium in the diet or stressful lifestyle"	"better awareness programs" "classes offered free to educate the masses" "education on healthier eating and the risk of habits that are dangerous to the body" "health seminars" "healthier restaurants in the area" "more free screenings from clinics"	• Racial and Ethnic Approaches to Community Health (REACH) policy, systems, and environmental change strategies—Healthy Corner Store Initiative • Community-funded grant to increase healthy lifestyles—*Weight Loss=Health Gain*
Diabetes (pre-, type 1, type 2)	"high sugar intake" "lack of good food choices" "poor eating habits" "stores without fresh produce"	"build better stores in the community with veggies" "eat healthy" "health class to inform the uninformed" "make healthier food selections available at local markets" "offer free exercise and cooking classes"	• Safe Routes to School Initiative Adaptation in RPC School (REACH) • Community health workers hired from RPC residents trained and supported in efforts to reduce/prevent and manage CVD and diabetes
HIV/AIDS	"having sex, sharing needles, blood to blood contact" "no awareness program" "unprotected sex"	"I wish I knew the answer . . . but a lot of things start with awareness and education" "people should be more informed about the spreading of HIV and prevention" "preventive classes" "safe sex"	• The MSM PRC core research project: A Multi-method Approach to STI and HIV/ AIDS Prevention among Urban Minority Youth—HIV/AIDS Prevention Program for Youth

CHNA processes that promoted success are listed below:

- Moving beyond documenting health disparities to advancing a health equity agenda requires an initial assessment of the health status of underserved populations (secondary data) and their own perceived health priorities, preferences, and experiences (primary data).
- The CBPR-driven CHNA process empowered community members to take on roles as researchers who develop locally relevant research questions and identify health disparities and determinants, thereby establishing processes and a research agenda rooted in community needs.
- The CHNA process allowed the MSM PRC to foster and expand relationships with the community in order to better understand and respond to its unique health priorities and capitalize on its strengths and assets.
- CHNA results, disseminated through community briefs and community conversations, serve as a resource through local data that can be used to inform neighborhood-driven community health action planning.

CBPR and the Atlanta/Georgia Clinical and Translational Science Awards

With translational and participatory models becoming essential to the national prevention research agenda, building of research capacity has been utilized to address power differentials between CBOs and researchers through CBPR. According to Wallerstein, building of research capacity is linked to health outcomes, in that skill development increases confidence and empowerment, which, in turn, generates community-owned health interventions that are more effective in improving health.[73] Partnership strategies for development of CBPR capacity have been evaluated through approaches ranging from qualitative stakeholder reflections to more rigorous, longitudinal designs.[16, 17, 73, 74]

The NIH-funded Clinical and Translational Science Award (CTSA) program was launched in 2006 and has expanded to over 50 academic medical institutions across the country. All funded CTSAs require a community engagement component, thus recognizing the important role it plays in translational research that leads to population health. The Atlanta Clinical and Translation Science Institute (ACTSI), now the Georgia CTSA, is an interinstitutional collaboration between Emory University, MSM, Georgia Institute of Technology, and its latest Georgia partner institution, the University of Georgia. ACTSI's Community Engagement Research Program (CERP) aimed to support community-university research partnerships, to facilitate community input into university research, and to increase health research in community settings that is both responsive and relevant to the health needs of the community. Both the ACTSI and the Georgia CTSA community engagement programs have been directed by the MSM PRC (2007–present), with co-directors at Emory University and the University of Georgia. The ACTSI-CERP is guided by a steering board, adopted from the MSM PRC CCB model, complete with a majority of its members from the community, rather than academic institutions. Community members are recruited from a variety of CBOs that are actively engaged in academic-community partnerships.

To date, 26 community-academic research partnered grants have been funded between 2008 and 2016, totaling $264,000. All grants were selected following submission of applications and peer review by a panel of community and academic leaders who produce scores and feedback based on standardized rubrics designed to assess innovation of the project and community engagement relevance. Grants were awarded to CBOs rather than academic faculty. Each awardee was required to have an academic research collaborator and to submit a final report. Each community and academic partner completed a key informant interview to discuss the experience. Projects funded over time have included those designed to (1) plan, implement, and evaluate health-related projects (Model 1); (2) facilitate community-led dissemination of academic research discoveries (Model 2); and (3) increase capacities in the conduct of community-engaged research (community and academic researchers) and toward implementation of a pilot research project (the Building

Collaborative Research Capacity Model [BCRCM]; Model 3). The BCRCM was developed through the ACTSI's CERP Building Collaborative Research Capacity Grant Program.[75] Collaborative research capacity is defined as the skills, values, and resources needed to engage all partners equitably in the full research process. Review of the literature and CBPR experience informed identification of domains of collaborative research capacity, including shared goals, attitudes toward collaboration, institutional factors, mutual respect, human and fiscal resources, partnering skills, and research skills. Table 3.4 defines each domain and implications for collaboration.[75]

Below are five recommendations from experiences in collaborating with CBOs and academic faculty to facilitate community-engaged research:[33]

Table 3.4 Domains for Building Collaborative Research Capacity Model

Domain	Definition	Implications for collaboration
Research skills	A set of skills required to carry out research, such as study design, instrument development, data analysis	Enhances partner equity and increases likelihood for future collaboration
Shared goals	Existence of common objectives and/or collaborative activities that contribute to sustaining the partnership	Project remains focused and partners share successes and failures
Attitudes toward collaboration	Attitudes and organizational cultures that encourage and support community-engaged research	Increases desired outcomes and sustained collaboration in the past
		Acknowledges potential negative experiences from collaboration in the past
Institutional factors	Factors existing in academic/CBO systems that encourage or hinder collaborative research	Challenges at the institutional level are recognized and addressed when feasible early in the research process
Mutual respect	Established rapport or sense of trust	Limits conflict by providing tangible benefits to each partner
Human and fiscal resources	The staff, monies, and space to carry out the research	Allocation of monies and resources impact partner equity and ability to carry out research tasks
Partnering skills	A set of skills required to work effectively with others, such as communication, dependability, and transparency	Opens channels of communication and builds trust among partners

1. Infuse ethics and IRB education specifically related to community-engaged research for both CBOs and their academic research partners.
2. Facilitate formal meetings and communication between CBOs and academic researchers as early as possible to cultivate communication regarding roles and ensure progress on the collaborative research.
3. Employ quantitative and qualitative methods to model processes and their linkages to associated research outcomes.
4. Facilitate technical support, with requirements delineated at program onset, as partners may be collaborating, formally, for the first time.
5. Establish outlets, identified by each partner, for promoting the academic-community partnership (i.e., grand rounds, seminars, workshops, websites, social media) for increased visibility and credibility with audiences that they value.

The Educational Program to Increase Colorectal Cancer Screening (EPICS)

The colorectal cancer mortality rate is about 40 percent higher in African Americans than in Whites. Most colorectal cancer deaths could be prevented by screening, but only about 60 percent of African Americans over age 50 (the recommended age for initiating screening) have been screened (Whites don't do much better).

In 2010, supported by a CDC grant, the MSM PRC demonstrated the efficacy of an educational intervention that was developed with the help of a community coalition called the Metropolitan Atlanta Coalition on Cancer Awareness. It was tested using a CBPR approach with the involvement of the MSM PRC CCB. The intervention brought a small group of unscreened African Americans together with a health educator for four one-hour sessions each a week apart. During the sessions, participants learned the risk factors for colorectal cancer and its clinical features; in addition, they learned about the types of screening tests and the importance of getting screened. Six months later, those participating in the intervention had a screening rate twice that of a control group that had only received literature about the disease (35% compared to 17%).[76]

But interventions that work well in a research setting often perform poorly in a "real-world" environment, where health promotion workers do not have research staff and the other advantages that a research grant has to offer. To test the intervention in practice, the MSM PRC partnered with the county health department to conduct the intervention in the county's 17 senior centers, using health department staff functioning under "usual" conditions. The health department's health educators felt that four sessions were excessive, so we condensed the material into three sessions. The outcome was almost exactly the same as it had been in the community intervention trial.[77]

We then submitted EPICS to the National Cancer Institute for publication on its Research-Tested Intervention Programs website (on the site it is labeled as "Colorectal Cancer Screening Intervention Program").[78] The site offers detailed instructions for cancer prevention interventions. After peer review, the intervention was accepted. We subsequently introduced EPICS to five of the state-sponsored Georgia Cancer Coalitions—regional organizations of health professionals and cancer advocates that promote cancer prevention.

A grant from the National Cancer Institute has enabled us to test EPICS at 20 sites around the country.[79] At these sites, the health educators and community health workers are volunteer members of community coalitions that were organized several years earlier by the National Black Leadership Initiative on Cancer, a National Cancer Institute–sponsored cancer prevention program. In this project, the intervention is being tested under varying circumstances to identify the best approach to training the health educators and CHWs. At this writing, results are being analyzed.

In summary, EPICS is an intervention designed to address a health disparity by a partnership between MSM and a community coalition. It was tested with a CBPR approach and was shown to be efficacious. Its efficacy was demonstrated in a practice setting. It has subsequently been used by a number of community coalitions.

The Next Research Frontier: Tˣ™—Advancing Translation to Transformation

The translational science spectrum consists of phases or types of research—from discoveries that advance our understanding of the biological basis of health and disease to interventions that engage individuals and social systems toward improved population health. The schematic depiction of translational research is often a series of "Ts" ("T" for translation stage) proceeding in order from T_0 to T_5 (with variations in the number of discrete stages identified). The path from observation and analysis of phenomena to real-world health impact can emanate from *any* of the T phases. According to NIH, translation is the process through which scientific discoveries (laboratory, clinic, and community, among others) advance improvements in the health of individuals or populations—"from diagnostics and therapeutics to medical procedures and behavioral changes."[80]

The heath research system has widely acknowledged flaws that delay (or even deny) the fruits of research findings for the population as a whole and for chronically disadvantaged groups in particular. Studies suggest that it takes an average of 17 years for some scientific discoveries to advance across the translation phases into practice.[81] This sluggishness can be significantly exacerbated among minority populations that experience the burden of the disease in question. A myriad of other interwoven variables, including, but not limited to, variations in population genetics, sociodemographic factors, environmental exposures, and systemic factors, may impede adoption of cutting-edge approaches for the populations in greatest need. This relative lack of participation in, for instance, pharmaceutical research may lead to a failure to identify differing therapeutic/toxicity profiles, unexpected allergy-inducing potential, or other concerns. The higher prevalence of these problems among some Blacks is usually interpreted by clinicians as a reason to avoid a certain drug class. While a higher prevalence of such problems is obviously concerning, the effect of large-scale avoidance of medications that actually may be good for most affected African Americans can result in a widening of health disparities. Health insurance challenges, other impediments to care access, and even the details of the provider-patient relationship can further degrade the opportunity for improving health outcomes.

Understanding this level of complexity and corresponding solutions is beyond the limited scope of any *single* translational research discipline or category along the translational (T_0-T_5) continuum. There is growing recognition of a need for new approaches and lenses through which to not only conduct collaborative research but also advance health equity through responsive interventions and programs tailored to the contexts of priority communities, practice, policy, and industry partners that are central to moving the proverbial needle. Efforts to accelerate chronic disease prevention and reduce health inequities are increasingly focused on policy, systems, and environmental change approaches. The CDC has highlighted the importance of coordination among multiple sectors as a key to successful efforts.[82] The National Academy of Medicine has further emphasized the importance of engaging the nonhealth sectors in changing policies and environments to address chronic disease.

We need more research and improved ways to *adopt* research discoveries to improve the health of populations. This will require a multiplicity of disciplines, perspectives, and interdisciplinary scientists (biomedical, sociocultural, and behavioral) in collaboration and characterized by systematic communication and iterative interaction. This ideally would allow discovery and the advancement gained in *any* phase of the "T" continuum to inform and enhance other phases of research or implementation.

T^x™: The Approach, Philosophy, and Scholarship

Coined at MSM, T^x™ symbolizes an approach and scientific philosophy that intentionally promotes and supports convergence of interdisciplinary research and scientists to stimulate exponential advances for the health of diverse communities. The "T" of the trademark acknowledges the importance of the phases of the translational continuum. However, the exponent "x" represents the goal to move research from the translational to the transformational. This research engages diverse disciplines and perspectives early in the process of identifying/framing the problem or opportunity. Further, it brings to bear different repositories of knowledge, skill, and lived experience.

What Is T^{x}™ Scholarship?

MSM T^{x}™ is a comprehensive approach and philosophy that advances the science, practice, and evaluation of improving health outcomes. It addresses disparities by simultaneously engaging multiple disciplines as it recognizes the multiple layers and dimensions of complex health problems. The aim of T^{x}™ is the advancement of health equity, which is the cornerstone of MSM's vision. T^{x}™ scholarship is characterized by the practices outlined below:

- *Engages multidisciplinary researchers across the translational continuum/rings (basic to population-based scientists) to work together toward the development, implementation, evaluation, and dissemination of innovative science.* Rubio and others have built on well-respected definitions of translational research, defining it as a discipline that involves the intentional collaboration of researchers along the T spectrum, thereby moving bidirectionally and in a multidisciplinary fashion.[81] In order to fully actualize this through a T^{x}™ scholarship lens, approaches to training, scholarship, and faculty promotion must foster and reward collaborative researchers that demonstrate how they capitalize on the exponential research innovations that emerge from cross-translational research.
- *Engages the community (patients and neighborhood residents) from the inception of research concept and/or identifies potential community needs, strengths, and implications/impact of research, through community-engaged research partnerships and collaborations or CBPR.*
- *Convenes interdisciplinary teams (which may include but is not limited to nonacademic industry, agency, and policy partners) to*

prioritize multilevel translation, dissemination, and proof-of-impact strategies associated with research and evaluation, encompassing both processes and outcomes. Transformative research that embodies T×™ research also engages other relevant stakeholders (nonacademic and beyond community residents and patients) pivotal to the uptake and adaptation of research findings in practice. Tabak et al. describe the relatively recent (15-year) evolution of implementation science.[83] These approaches infuse research into practice by integrating practitioners into research evaluation (so-called practice-based evidence). This expanded approach to team science includes practice partners (clinical, industry, public health leaders) from the inception and conceptualization of research development and facilitates adopting research findings in the real world, rather than in a controlled research setting.

- *Includes adoption and/or adaptation to communities of (1) those who are underserved/at risk/vulnerable, (2) science, and (3) practice (clinical, public health, policy) based on cooperative needs.* Collaboration should involve people or organizations from multiple sectors (e.g., planners, developers, media specialists, neighborhood residents, elected officials) and geographical strata (e.g., state, regional, local, neighborhood). Collaborative groups that promote stakeholder engagement and interaction have been associated with increased relevance, feasibility, and long-term sustainability of initiatives.[84] These groups have the potential to develop and maintain strategies to increase opportunities by leveraging resources, sharing knowledge, and building relationships that advance the translation of evidence-based research in communities of practice, where health system transformation can occur.[84, 85]

- *Finally, MSM T×™ scholarship is a practice and philosophy that leads the conduct of research with results that broaden the evidence base through data-driven proof of impact on health equity in underserved or special populations.* The rigor of research is not diminished through conducting T×™ scholarship. In fact, the evidence of effectiveness of both practice-based research and research-based practice is heightened given their joint implications for laboratory, bedside, and community research and real-world impact. The sound conduct of research that advances discoveries in each discrete T phase through traditional investigator-initiated science therefore *must* be conducted in parallel with more collaborative T^{xTM} research scholarship. It is imperative, however, that as definitions of vulnerable populations and those with health disparities expand and contract with local, regional, and global priorities, research is both translational and transformative in response. Our collective responsiveness to obstinate and emerging health disparities, with their multilevel and complex fundamental causes, must be met by equally integrated approaches.

MSM institutionally invested in the inaugural T^{xTM} pilot projects program led by multidisciplinary basic, clinical, and social behavioral researchers in 2018. The vision of MSM is *to lead the creation and advancement of health equity.* Health equity is a destination that will ensure that "every person has the opportunity to 'attain his or her full health potential' and no one is 'disadvantaged from achieving this potential because of social position or other socially determined circumstances.'"[86] These advances require the contributions of disciplines beyond the "bench and bedside" and may include health services, CBPR, or population-based approaches that consider lifestyle and behavior modification strategies. This evidence base must then be applied and associated with the adoption of interventions into routine patient and population health care. T^{xTM} is therefore a destination that is ever evolving and is responsive to the research, the needs of priority populations, and collaboration with partners in order to transform health, thereby advancing health equity.[87]

Summary

The CBPR philosophy is one designed to advance not only rigorous research but practically significant approaches that address social injustice through policy, systems, and environmental change. It is not one designed solely to create goodwill between community residents and academic partners toward improving research recruitment and retention. It is based on attention toward development and seeding of relationships based on mutual benefit and synergies. This requires attention to historical power differentials through systems and processes that prioritize community elevation and trust, thereby emphasizing not only statistically significance research but also the dynamics and relative strength of the partnership. The exemplars detailed in this chapter described how the CE effort stimulated by the Morehouse Model has morphed into a community-based approach for research on health disparities to advance health equity.

References

1. "Health Equity and Social Justice." Boston Public Health Commission. http://www.bphc.org/whatwedo/health-equity-social-justice/Pages/Health-Equity-and -Social-Justice.aspx.

2. "National Institute on Minority Health and Heath Disparities." US Department of Health and Human Services. https://www.nimhd.nih.gov/about/overview/.

3. "Healthy People 2020." US Department of Health and Human Services, Office of Disease Prevention and Health Promotion. https://www.healthypeople.gov/2020 /topics-objectives/topic/social-determinants-of-health.

4. Centers for Disease Control and Prevention. 2013. "CDC Health Disparities and Inequalities Report." *MMWR* 62 (Suppl. 3): 3–5.

5. Oetzel, J. G., et al. 2018. "Impact of Participatory Health Research: A Test of the Community-Based Participatory Research Conceptual Model." *BioMed Research International* 2018:7281405. doi:10.1155/2018/7281405.

6. McOliver, C. A., A. K. Camper, J. T. Doyle, M. J. Eggers, T. E. Ford, M. A. Lila, J. Berner, L. Campbell, and J. Donatuto. 2015. "Community Based Research as a Mechanism to Reduce Environmental Health Disparities in American Indian and Alaska Native Communities." *International Journal of Environmental Research and Public Health* 12 (4): 4076–4100.

7. Case, A. D., et al. 2014. "Stakeholders' Perspectives on Community-Based Participatory Research to Enhance Mental Health Services." *American Journal of Community Psychology* 54 (3–4): 397–408.

8. Jagosh, J., et al. 2012. "Uncovering the Benefits of Participatory Research: Implications of a Realist Review for Health Research and Practice." *Milbank Quarterly* 90 (2): 311–46.

9. Cargo, M., and S. L. Mercer. 2008. "The Value and Challenges of Participatory Research: Strengthening Its Practice." *Annual Review of Public Health* 29:325–50.

10. Israel, B. A., E. Eng, A. J. Schulz, and E. A. Parker. 2005. *Methods in Community-Based Participatory Research for Health*. San Francisco: Jossey-Bass.

11. Akintobi, T. H., et al. 2018. "Processes and Outcomes of a Community-Based Participatory Research-Driven Health Needs Assessment: A Tool for Moving Health Disparity Reporting to Evidence-Based Action." *Progress in Community Health Partnerships: Research, Education, and Action* 12 (1S): 139–47.

12. Blumenthal, D. S. 2006. "A Community Coalition Board Creates a Set of Values for Community-Based Research." *Preventing Chronic Disease* 3 (1): A16.

13. Wallerstein, Nina, Bonnie Duran, John G. Oetzel, and Meredith Minkler, eds. 2018. *Community-Based Participatory Research for Health: Advancing Social and Health Equity*. 3rd ed. San Francisco: Jossey-Bass.

14. Israel, Barbara A., Eugenia Eng, Amy J. Schulz, and Edith A. Parker, eds. 2012. *Methods for Community-Based Participatory Research for Health*. 2nd ed. San Francisco: Jossey-Bass.

15. Dankwa-Mullan, I., K. B. Rhee, K. Williams, I. Sanchez, F. S. Sy, N. Stinson Jr., and J. Ruffin. 2010. "The Science of Eliminating Health Disparities: Summary and Analysis of the NIH Summit Recommendations." *American Journal of Public Health* 100 (Suppl. 1): S12–18.

16. Allen, M., K. Culhane-Pera, S. Pergament, and T. Call. 2011. "A Capacity Building Program to Promote CBPR Partnerships between Academic Researchers and Community Members." *Clinical and Translational Science* 4 (6): 428–33.

17. Tendulkar, S. A., J. Chu, J. Opp, A. Geller, A. Digirolamo, E. Gandelman, M. Grullon, P. Patil, S. King, and K. Hacker. 2011. "A Funding Initiative for Community-Based Participatory Research: Lessons from the Harvard Catalyst Seed Grants." *Progress in Community Health Partnerships* 5 (1): 35–44.

18. Balas, E. A., and S. A. Boren. 2000. "Managing Clinical Knowledge for Healthcare Improvement." In *Yearbook of Medical Informatics 2000: Patient-Centered Systems*, ed. J. Bemmel and A. T. McCray. Stuttgart: Schattauer Verlagsgesellschaft.

19. Glasgow, R. E., E. Lichtenstein, and A. C. Marcus. 2003. "Why Don't We See More Translation of Health Promotion Research to Practice? Rethinking the Efficacy-to-Effectiveness Transition." *American Journal of Public Health* 93 (8): 1261–67.

20. Staniszewska, S., K. L. Haywood, J. Brett, and L. Tutton. 2012. "Patient and Public Involvement in Developing Patient-Reported Outcome Measures: Evolution Not Revolution." *Patient* 5 (2): 79–87.

21. Park, Jinbin. 2017. "Historical Origins of the Tuskegee Experiment: The Dilemma of Public Health in the United States." *Korean Journal of Medical History* 26 (3): 545–78. doi:10.13081/kjmh.2017.26.545.

22. Kerpel-Fronius, Sándor. 2008. "The Epoch-Changing Influence of the Nuremberg Doctor's Trial on the Ethical Judgment of Human Experiments." *Orvosi Hetilap* 149 (5): 195–201. doi:10.1556/OH.2008.28282.

23. Jones, Bridgette L., Carrie A. Vyhlidal, Andrea Bradley-Ewing, Ashley Sherman, and Kathy Goggin. 2017. "If We Would Only Ask: How Henrietta Lacks Continues to Teach Us about Perceptions of Research and Genetic Research among African Americans Today." *Journal of Racial and Ethnic Health Disparities* 4 (4): 735–45. doi:10.1007/s40615-016-0277-1.

24. Wallerstein, N., and B. Duran. 2010. "Community-Based Participatory Research Contributions to Intervention Research: The Intersection of Science and Practice to Improve Health Equity." *American Journal of Public Health* 100 (S1): S40–46.

25. Blumenthal, D. 2011. "How Do You Start Working with a Community?" In *Principles of Community Engagement*, 2nd ed., by Clinical and Translational Science Awards Consortium Community Engagement Key Function Committee Task Force on the Principles of Community Engagement, 134–35. Washington, DC: US Department of Health and Human Services.

26. Akintobi Henry, T., L. Goodin, E. Heard Trammel, D. Collins, and D. Blumenthal. 2011. "How Do You Set Up and Maintain a Community Advisory Board?" In *Principles of Community Engagement*, 2nd ed., by Clinical and Translational Science Awards Consortium Community Engagement Key Function Committee Task Force on the Principles of Community Engagement, 136–38. Washington, DC: US Department of Health and Human Services.

27. Akintobi, T. H., N. Dawood, and D. S. Blumenthal. 2014. "An Academic–Public Health Department Partnership for Education, Research, Practice and Governance." *Journal of Public Health Management and Practice* 20 (3): 310–14.

28. Akintobi, T. H., L. Goodin, and L. Hoffman. 2013. "Morehouse School of Medicine Prevention Research Center: Collaborating with Neighborhoods to Develop Community-Based Participatory Approaches to Address Health Disparities in Metropolitan Atlanta." *Atlanta Medicine: Journal of the Medical Association of Atlanta* 84 (2): 14–17.

29. Akintobi, T. H., E. Lockamy, L. Goodin, N. Hernandez, T. Slocumb, D. Blumenthal, and L. Hoffman. 2018. "Processes and Outcomes of a Community-Based Participatory Research-Driven Health Needs Assessment: A Tool for Moving Health Disparity Reporting to Evidence-Based Action." *Progress in Community Health Partnerships: Research, Education, and Action* 12 (1S): 139–47. doi:10.1353/cpr.2018.0029.

30. Moodley, K., T. H. Akintobi, T. Fish, and D. Blumenthal. 2018. "A Pipeline Program to Address the African Crisis in Human Resources for Health." *Annals of Global Health* 84 (1): 66–76.

31. Gaglioti, A., X. Junjun, L. Rollins, P. Baltrus, K. O'Connell, D. Cooper, and T. H. Akintobi. 2018. "Neighborhood Environmental Health and Premature Cardiovascular Death in Atlanta: A Secondary Data Analysis Motivated by Community Wisdom from the REACH Project." *Preventing Chronic Disease* 15 (17): 1–12. doi:10.5888/pcd15.170220.

32. Hoffman, L. M., L. Rollins, T. H. Akintobi, K. Erwin, K. Lewis, N. Hernandez, and A. Miller. 2017. "Oral Health Intervention for Low-Income African American Men in Atlanta, Georgia." *American Journal of Public Health* 107 (S1): S104–10. doi:10.2105/AJPH.2017.303760.

33. Akintobi, T. H., D. E. Wilkerson, K. Rodgers, C. Escoffery, R. Haardörfer, and M. Kegler. 2016. "Assessment of the Building Collaborative Research Capacity Model: Bridging the Community-Academic Researcher Divide." *Journal of the Georgia Public Health Association* 6 (2): 123–32.

34. Zellner, T., T. H. Akintobi, A. Miller, E. Archie-Booker, T. Johnson, and D. Evans. 2016. "Assessment of a Culturally Tailored Sexual Health Education Program for African American Youth." *International Journal of Environmental Research and Public Health* 14 (1): 14. doi:10.3390/ijerph14010014.

35. Caplan, L., T. H. Akintobi, T. Gordon, T. Zellner, S. Smith, and D. Blumenthal. 2016. "Reducing Disparities by Way of a Cancer Disparities Research Training Program." *Journal of Health Disparities Research and Practice* 9 (3): 103–14.

36. Walls, C., T. H. Akintobi, R. Willock, A. Miller, J. Trotter, and S. Lenoir. 2016. "Impact of Perceived Stress on Alcohol, Substance Abuse and Risky Sexual Behavior among Black Women 18 to 24 Years of Age in Urban Neighborhoods." *International Journal of Ethnic College Health* 2 (1): 19–27.

37. Akintobi, T. H., N. Laster, J. Trotter, D. Jacobs, T. Johnson, T. King Gordon, and A. Miller. 2016. "The Health, Enlightenment, Awareness, and Living (HEAL) Intervention: Outcome of an HIV and Hepatitis B and C Risk Reduction Intervention." *International Journal of Environmental Research and Public Health* 13 (10): 948.

38. Holliday, R. C., R. Braithwaite, E. Yancey, T. Akintobi, D. Stevens-Watkins, S. Smith, and C. Powell. 2016. "Substance Use Correlates of Depression among African American Male Inmates, Public Health and Incarceration: Social Justice Matters." *Journal of Healthcare for the Poor and Underserved* 27 (2A): 181–93.

39. Akintobi, T. H., J. Trotter, T. Zellner, S. Lenoir, D. Evans, L. Rollins, and A. Miller. 2016. "Outcomes of a Behavioral Intervention to Increase Condom Use and Reduce HIV Risk among Urban African American Young Adults." *Health Promotion Practice* 17 (5): 751–59.

40. Akintobi, T. H., L. Hoffman, C. McAllister, L. Goodin, N. Hernandez, L. Rollins, and A. Miller. 2016. "Assessing the Oral Health Needs of Black Men in Low-Income, Urban Communities." *American Journal of Men's Health* 12 (2): 326–37.

41. Bolar, C., N. Hernandez, T. H. Akintobi, C. McAllister, A. Ferguson, L. Rollins, and T. Clem. 2016. "Context Matters: A Community-Based Study of Urban Minority Parents' Views on Child Health." *Journal of the Georgia Public Health Association* 5 (3): 212–19.

42. Kegler, M., D. Blumenthal, T. H. Akintobi, K. Rodgers, K. Erwin, W. Thompson, and E. Hopkins. 2016. "Lessons Learned from Three Models That Use Small Grants for Building Academic-Community Partnerships for Research." *Journal of Health Care for the Poor and the Underserved* 27 (2): 527–48.

43. Yancey, R., R. Mayberry, E. Armstrong-Mensah, D. Collins, L. Goodin, S. Cureton, E. H. Trammell, and K. Yuan. 2003. "The Community-Based Participatory Intervention Effect of 'HIV-RAAP.'" *American Journal of Health Behavior* 36 (4): 555–68.

44. Zellner, T., T. Trotter, S. Lenoir, K. Walston, L. Men-Na'a, T. Henry-Akintobi, and A. Miller. 2015. "Color It Real: A Program to Increase Condom Use and Reduce Substance Abuse and Perceived Stress." *International Journal of Environmental Research and Public Health* 13 (1): 51.

45. Sufian, M., J. Grunbaum, T. Akintobi, A. Dozier, M. Eder, S. Jones, and S. White-Cooper. 2011. "Program Evaluation and Evaluating Community Engagement." In *Principles of Community Engagement*, 2nd ed., by Clinical and Translational Science Award Community Engagement Key Function Committee Task Force on the Principles of Community Engagement, 163–82. Washington, DC: US Department of Health and Human Services.

46. Akintobi, T., K. Holden, L. Rollins, R. Lyn, H. Heiman, P. Daniels, and L. Hoffman. 2016. "Applying a Community-Based Participatory Research Approach to Address Determinants of Cardiovascular Disease and Diabetes Mellitus in an Urban Setting." In *Handbook of Community-Based Participatory Research*, ed. S. Coughlin, S. Smith, and M. Fernandez, 131–54. New York: Oxford University Press.

47. Akintobi, T. H., R. Braithwaite, and A. Dodds. 2014. "Residential Segregation: Trends and Implications for Conducting Effective Community-Based Research

to Address Ethnic Health Disparities." In *Uprooting Urban America: Multidisciplinary Perspectives on Race, Class and Gentrification*, ed. H. Hall, C. Cole-Robinson, and A. Kohli, 157–69. New York: Peter Lang.

48. "Neighborhood Planning Unit (NPU)." City of Atlanta, GA. www.atlantaga.gov/index.aspx?page=739.

49. City of Atlanta, Department of Planning and Community Development Office of Planning. 2010. *Census Summary Report Neighborhood Planning Unit V*. www.atlantaga.gov/modules/showdocument.aspx?documentid=3897.

50. City of Atlanta, Department of Planning and Community Development Office of Planning. 2010. *Census Summary Report Neighborhood Planning Unit X*. www.atlantaga.gov/modules/showdocument.aspx?documentid=3895.

51. City of Atlanta, Department of Planning and Community Development Office of Planning. 2010. *Census Summary Report Neighborhood Planning Unit Y*. www.atlantaga.gov/modules/showdocument.aspx?documentid=3894.

52. City of Atlanta, Department of Planning and Community Development Office of Planning. 2010. *Census Summary Report Neighborhood Planning Unit Z*. www.atlantaga.gov/modules/showdocument.aspx?documentid=3893.

53. Georgia Institute of Technology Center for Geographic Information Systems. 2013. *Atlanta Neighborhood Quality of Life and Health 2013*. Atlanta: Georgia Institute of Technology. https://cspav.gatech.edu/NQOLH/Project/.

54. Lee, S., and S. Guhathakurta. 2013. "Bridging Environmental Sustainability and Quality of Life in Metropolitan Atlanta's Urban Communities." In *Community Quality-of-Life Indicators: Best Cases VI*, ed. M. J. Sirgy, R. Phillips, and D. Rahtz, 207–31. New York: Springer.

55. "Mortality." Georgia Department of Public Health, Office of Health Indicators for Planning. https://oasis.state.ga.us/oasis/webquery/qryMortality.aspx.

56. Blumenthal, D. S. 2001. "Is Community-Based Participatory Research Possible?" *American Journal of Preventive Medicine* 40 (3): 386–89.

57. Bringle, R. G., and J. A. Hatcher. 2002. "Campus-Community Partnerships: The Terms of Engagement." *Journal of Social Issues* 58 (3): 503–16.

58. Andrews, J. O., G. Bentley, S. Crawford, L. Pretlow, and M. S. Tingen. 2007. "Using Community-Based Participatory Research to Develop a Culturally Sensitive Smoking Cessation Intervention with Public Housing Neighborhoods." *Ethnicity and Disease* 17 (2): 331–37.

59. Newman, S. D., J. O. Andrews, G. S. Magwood, C. Jenkins, M. J. Cox, and D. C. Williamson. 2011. "Community Advisory Boards in Community-Based Participatory Research: A Synthesis of Best Processes." *Preventing Chronic Disease* 8 (3): A70.

60. Homans, G. C. 1961. *Social Behavior*. New York: Harcourt Brace & World.

61. Thibaut, J. W., and H. H. Kelley. 1959. *The Social Psychology of Groups*. New York: Wiley.

62. Hatch, J., N. Moss, A. Saran, and L. Presley-Cantrell. 1993. "Community Research: Partnership in Black Communities." *American Journal of Preventive Medicine* 9 (6): 27–31.

63. Commission on Social Determinants of Health. 2008. *Closing the Gap in a Generation: Health Equity through Action on the Social Determinants of Health*. Final Report of the Commission on Social Determinants of Health. Geneva: World Health Organization.

64. Hebert-Beirne, J., J. K. Felner, Y. Castañeda, and S. Cohen. 2017. "Enhancing Themes and Strengths Assessment: Leveraging Academic-Led Qualitative Inquiry in Community Health Assessment to Uncover Roots of Community Health Inequities." *Journal of Public Health Management and Practice* 23 (4): 370–79.

65. Ainsworth, D., H. Diaz, and M. C. Schmidtlein. 2012. "Getting More for Your Money." *Health Promotion Practice* 14 (6): 868–75.

66. Cain, C. L., D. Orionzi, M. O'Brien, and L. Trahan. 2016. "The Power of Community Voices for Enhancing Community Health Needs Assessments." *Health Promotion Practice* 18 (3): 437–43.

67. Black, K. Z., C. Y. Hardy, M. De Marco, A. S. Ammerman, G. Corbie-Smith, B. Council, and A. Lightfoot. 2013. "Beyond Incentives for Involvement to Compensation for Consultants: Increasing Equity in CBPR Approaches." *Progress in Community Health Partnerships* 7 (3): 263–70.

68. Srinivasan, S., and G. W. Collman. 2005. "Evolving Partnerships in Community." *Environmental Health Perspectives* 113 (12): 1814–16.

69. Israel, B. A., A. J. Schulz, E. A. Parker, and A. B. Becker. 2001. "Community-Based Participatory Research: Policy Recommendations for Promoting a Partnership Approach in Health Research." *Education for Health* 14 (2): 182–97.

70. Israel, B. A., A. J. Schulz, E. A. Parker, and A. B. Becker. 1998. "Review of Community-Based Research: Assessing Partnership Approaches to Improve Public Health." *Annual Review of Public Health* 19:173–202.

71. Jones, L., B. Meade, N. Forge, M. Moini, F. Jones, C. Terry, and K. Norris. "Begin Your Partnership: The Process of Engagement." *Ethnicity and Disease* 19 (4 Suppl. 6): S6–8.16.

72. Suarez-Balcazar, Y., G. W. Harper, and R. Lewis. 2005. "An Interactive and Contextual Model of Community-University Collaborations for Research and Action." *Health Education and Behavior* 32 (1): 84–101.

73. Rollins, L., T. H. Akintobi, A. Hermstad, D. Cooper, L. Goodin, J. Beane, and R. Lyn. 2017. "Community-Based Approaches to Reduce Chronic Disease Disparities in Georgia." *Journal of the Georgia Public Health Association* 6 (4): 402–10. https://doi.org/10.21633/jgpha.6.403.

74. Wallerstein, N. B., and B. Duran. 2006. "Using Community-Based Participatory Research to Address Health Disparities." *Health Promotion Practice* 7 (3): 312–23.

75. Rogers, K., T. Akintobi, W. Thompson, C. Escoffery, D. Evans, and M. Kegler. 2014. "A Model for Strengthening Collaborative Research Capacity: Illustrations from the Atlanta Clinical Translational Science Institute." *Health Education and Behavior* 41 (3): 267–74. PMID:24311741.

76. Blumenthal, D. S., S. A. Smith, C. D. Majett, and E. Alema-Mensah. 2010. "A Trial of Three Interventions to Promote Colorectal Cancer Screening in African Americans." *Cancer* 116 (4): 922–29.

77. Smith, S. A., L. Johnson, D. Wesley, K. B. Turner, G. McCray, J. Sheats, and D. Blumenthal. 2012. "Translation to Practice of an Intervention to Promote Colorectal Cancer Screening among African Americans." *Clinical and Translational Science* 5 (5): 412–15.

78. "Colorectal Cancer Screening Intervention Program." National Cancer Institute. https://rtips.cancer.gov/rtips/programDetails.do?programId=1124686.

79. Smith, S. A., and D. S. Blumenthal. 2013. "Efficacy to Effectiveness Transition of an Educational Program to Increase Colorectal Cancer Screening (EPICS): Study Protocol of a Cluster Randomized Controlled Trial." *Implementation Science* 8:86.

80. National Center for Advancing Translational Science. 2015. *Translational Science Spectrum*. https://ncats.nih.gov/files/translation-factsheet.pdf.

81. Morris, Z. S., S. Wooding and J. Grant. 2011. "The Answer Is 17 Years, What Is the Question: Understanding Time Lags in Translational Research." *Journal of the Royal Society of Medicine* 104 (12): 510–20.

82. "Definition of Policy." Centers for Disease Control and Prevention, Office of the Associate Director for Policy. https://www.cdc.gov/policy/analysis/process /definition.html.

83. Tabak, R. G., E. C. Khoong, D. A. Chambers, and R. C. Brownson. 2012. "Bridging Research and Practice: Models for Dissemination and Implementation Research." *American Journal of Preventive Medicine* 43 (3): 337–50.

84. Wallerstein, N., and B. Duran. 2010. "Community-Based Participatory Research Contributions to Intervention Research: The Intersection of Science and Practice to Improve Health Equity." *American Journal of Public Health* 100 (S1): S40–46.

85. Tabak, R. G., M. M. Padek, J. F. Kerner, K. C. Stange, E. K. Proctor, M. J. Dobbins, and R. C. Brownson. 2017. "Dissemination and Implementation Science Training Needs: Insights from Practitioners and Researchers." *American Journal of Preventive Medicine* 52 (3): S322–29.

86. "Health Equity." Centers for Disease Control and Prevention, National Center for Chronic Disease Prevention and Health Promotion (NCCDPHP). https://www .cdc.gov/chronicdisease/healthequity/index.htm.

87. Henry Akintobi, T., J. Hopkins, K. Holden, D. Hefner, and H. Taylor. 2019. "TxTM: An Approach and Philosophy to Advance Translation to Transformation." *Ethnicity and Disease* 29 (Suppl. 2): 349–54. doi:10.18865/ed.29.S2.349.

FOUR

Evolution of the Morehouse Model for Community Engagement

I T IS "a marathon and not a sprint" when an institution's mission remains constant over four decades. This is true of Morehouse School of
Medicine's commitment to primary care and its commitment to engaging
disenfranchised and marginalized populations, wherever they are found.
Historically Black colleges and universities typically have constrained
human and fiscal resources when contrasted with predominantly White
institutions of higher education. HBCUs are challenged with having to do
more with less. Despite this observation, many of these institutions have
risen to prominence and excellence when you consider that HBCUs produce the most Black alumni who receive doctorates in science and engineering.[1] MSM has been on the receiving end of many HBCU feeder undergraduate programs that enable MSM to enroll some of the best and
the brightest students in our health professions program.

HBCUs have traditionally functioned as a magnet for Black students
at all levels nationwide and have advanced mentorship for preparing
young researchers in many fields.[2] These young investigators are usually equipped with a multicultural orientation, which better prepares
them to be of service to all client populations irrespective of race, gender, or sexual orientation. This is true largely owing to the cultural competencies highlighted at these institutions, and definitely at MSM. Having cultural competence is critical to effective community engagement.

The interpersonal skills required to effectively interface with community residents from low-income urban and rural areas is highlighted in our Community Health and Preventive Medicine Residency Program and in the many community-based participatory research programs implemented since the school's inception. Many of these (CBPR) programs have targeted both rural and urban neighborhoods as intervention sites.

Urban and inner-city areas continue to be the bedrock of health disparities and are areas typically defined as having high density, nonagricultural work, and a large number of physical structures. These urban areas have characteristics that expose residents to health risks related to their living conditions. Contemporary scientists have identified structural impediments as social determinants of health. Hence, the lack of employment opportunities, substandard housing, poor quality of education, violence in the community, voter suppression, and other negative forces all serve to disempower and deauthorize citizens from the benefits of the "Great Society." While MSM has built its reputation on both rural and urban health interventions, its footprint in the Atlanta, Georgia, area has established how citizen engagement can change cultural norms and group behavior. The manifestation of this work vis-à-vis the Morehouse Model has spanned 40 years. This work is exemplified through a legacy of extramural programs funded by local, state, federal, and private sector grantors. This work has focused on community-perceived and community-driven concerns based on epidemiologic findings in cancer, substance abuse, mental health, cardiovascular diseases, crime and violence, HIV, and many other disease entities.

Table 4.1 provides a list of grant-funded projects of the Department of Community Health and Preventative Medicine in which CE was a central component of project implementation. The table also depicts the year(s) of funding, project title, funding source, award amount, urban versus rural emphasis, nature of coalition membership (consumer or agency dominated), and structure of the coalition (governance or advisory). To further elucidate the sustained evolution of the Morehouse Model implementations in both rural and urban areas, table 4.1 details and tracks many of the efforts to embrace CE and community-linked coalitions for health equity.

Table 4.1 List of Grants Involving the Use of Community Coalitions

Year(s)	Title	Agency	Amount	Urban/rural	Consumer-dominated coalition	Structure governance or advisory
1984–2017	**Area Health Education Center Program**	Health Resources and Services Administration	$12,697,709	Urban & Rural	No	Governance & Advisory
	AHEC is a "pipeline" program to improve access to high-quality health care in underserved rural and inner-city communities. Funds flow from the federal government to the medical school and then, through subcontracts, to independent Area Health Education Centers. Those centers are responsible for recruiting K–12 and college students into health professions training programs, for providing portions of their training in underserved communities, and for supporting practices in underserved communities through continuing education, library access, and other services. Morehouse School of Medicine housed the AHEC Program office, which had an Advisory Committee composed primarily of representatives of health professions schools that participated in the program, as well as the directors of the centers. Each center, which is a nonprofit corporation, has a board of directors, which is a governing board. The Board of Directors is a community coalition that includes representatives of local hospitals, health professions training programs, medical practices, and public agencies, as well as consumers.					
1986–91	**Avoidable Mortality from Cancer in Black Populations**	National Cancer Institute	$1,400,000	Urban	Yes	Governance
	This was a research program designed to test an in-home educational intervention to promote breast and cervical cancer screening among African American women. It was conducted through a partnership between MSM and the National Black Women's Health Project (now called the Black Women's Health Imperative), a nonprofit consumer organization that was based in Atlanta at that time. The NBWHP served a governance function. Its membership consisted primarily of health-conscious African American laywomen, as well as some health professionals.					
1987–97	**Health Promotion Resource Center**	Kaiser Family Foundation	$1,450,000	Urban & Rural	Yes	Advisory
	The HPRC, initially founded in 1987, was originally a partnership between MSM and the General Missionary Baptist Convention of Georgia (GMBCG). The partnership was composed of citizens, church leaders, and pastors from the Atlanta and Waycross area. Within these two sites community organization methods were employed to launch community needs assessments and subsequently health education programs in teen pregnancy and substance abuse education. The partnerships made use of frequent bilateral consultation sessions between HPRC staff at MSM and community organizers working for the GMBCG who were funded by the Kaiser Foundation. This initiative served as the nucleus for many subsequent faith-based health-oriented initiatives that were birthed on a regional level following the initial two years of planning implementations.					
1989–92	**A Three-Tier Implementation Proposal in Support of the Health Promotion Resource Center**	Kaiser Family Foundation	$1,005,000	Rural	Yes	Governance
	In 1989 the Kaiser Family Foundation funded MSM-HPRC to implement a train the trainer application of the Morehouse Model training at the county level. This initiative was identified as the Jim Alley Training Program. Jim Alley was the recently deceased state health department director. Each county subsequently developed a coalition and health education and health promotion projects consistent with the guidelines of the Morehouse Model. The coalitions were consumer dominated.					

1989–94	**Joyland/High Point Community Coalition Inc. CSAP High-Risk Youth**	Center for Substance Abuse Prevention	$1,000,000	Urban	Yes	Governance

In 1989, The Federal Center for Substance Abuse Prevention (CSAP) funded a coalition application submitted by MSM and a community-based organization (CBO) in urban Atlanta identified as the Joyland/High Point Coalition. Its membership was composed of community leaders, the principals of the local middle and high schools, law enforcement personnel, a pastor, two representatives from the local health department, a housing authority representative, four youth, and six local community residents. The coalition staff was funded with a subcontract from MSM. The mission of this initiative was to engage high school students in a substance abuse prevention mentoring program based on Afrocentric principles. High school students were trained as mentors to deliver a curriculum to 400 middle school students over a three-year period. Evaluated results indicated that the project was effective in improving academic performance and reducing disciplinary problems.

1989–93	**Project SUCCESS (Successful Utilization of a Community Coalition Empowered with Skills and Services)**	Federal Center for Substance Abuse Prevention	$231,000	Urban	Yes	Advisory

This initiative was directed toward low-income residents of a public housing complex (John Hope Franklin Housing Complex). A community coalition advisory board was organized, composed of the director of the local YMCA, law enforcement, public housing, a retired convenience store owner, a pastor, and eight residents from the Housing Complex. The charge to the coalition was to develop and implement an after-school health education program to teach critical thinking skills. The coalition made use of the Botvin Life Skills Model. The evidence-based substance abuse and violence prevention program is taught two to three times a week over an eight-week period. We exposed 120 residents to the training, and evaluation results showed sustained effects in reduced drug use by 25%, alcohol use by 60%, physical violence and aggression by 50%, and tobacco use by 87%.

1990–2005	**Health Education Training Centers**	Health Resources and Services Administration	$5,637,256	Rural	Yes	Governance & Advisory

This was a federally funded program in which the AHEC program participated. It provided the same services as the AHEC program with the addition of community organization and development for health promotion. This service was primarily provided by community health workers employed by the AHEC centers. The Program Office's Advisory Committee and the Centers' Board of Directors were the same as in the AHEC Program.

1990–94	**Rural Empowerment Coalitions for Long-Range Approaches to Inside Management (Project RECLAIM)**	Federal Center for Substance Abuse Prevention	$1,321,788	Rural	Yes	Governance

Project RECLAIM involved 10 rural coalitions funded for three years with the primary goal of preventing drug use in 10 rural Georgia counties. Each coalition included representation from media, faith, social services, education, law enforcement, local government, private industry, and community residents. Training was provided to each coalition in the Morehouse Model. During the coalition development stage, the 10 counties indicated that their greatest need was community mobilization strategies and methods for identifying and implementing substance abuse prevention programs. These coalitions also identified cancer screening and HIV prevention as important health planning areas.

(continued)

Table 4.1 (continued)

Year(s)	Title	Agency	Amount	Urban/rural	Consumer-dominated coalition	Structure governance or advisory
1990–96	**Community Partnership for Alcohol, Tobacco, and Other Drugs (ATOD)**	Center for Substance Abuse—SAMHSA	$1,800,000	Urban	No	Advisory

ATOD was a national program of 250 grantees serving communities throughout the nation. The Morehouse project organized an advisory coalition composed of 10 mandated partners representing education, housing, health, media, recreation, law enforcement, business, human services, and civic and faith communities. The coalition made use of several strategies to reach inner-city community residents with a prevention program. These included (1) community-wide education through media and public service announcements, (2) alternative and recreational activities for youth, (3) school-based prevention efforts, (4) workplace ATOD prevention, (5) youth employment, (6) technical assistance to CBOs and community groups, (7) provision of development funds for CBOs, and (8) cultural/ethnic events. The initiative was evaluated as part of a national evaluation. Results showed that gains were made in ATOD prevention behavior.

| 1990–96 | **Project MARTIN (Mentoring Adolescents for Risk Reduction through Training, Insulation and Nurturing)** | Center for Substance Abuse Prevention; The Department of Health and Human Services | $1,900,000 | Urban | Yes | Governance |

Project MARTIN was an adolescent substance abuse and family-life education program designed to educate students from Martin Luther King Jr. Middle School on the dangers of substance abuse and unprotected sex. A community coalition board was organized to use aspects of the Morehouse Model. The coalition was composed of six residents, four teens, two pastors, a high school principal, a middle school principal, a health department official, a housing department staffer, a radio media person, and two college students. This coalition became incorporated and convened on a monthly basis.

| 1987–92 | **Improving Community Health through Leadership Empowerment and Partnership** | W. K. Kellogg Foundation | $6,000,000 | Urban | Yes | Governance |

MSM coordinated the development of three urban community coalitions; two were in the city of Atlanta, and the third was in Kennesaw, Georgia. Each coalition was organized with local residents as the dominant members, although human service organizations (health, education, housing, recreation, faith) had a seat at the table as well. These coalitions were exposed to the Morehouse Model methodology beginning with community problem identification and needs assessment. They subsequently developed health education intervention programs to address selected community-documented health issues (teen pregnancy, violence, substance abuse, and sexually transmitted infections). The coalitions met on a monthly basis.

| 1993–96 | **Health of the Public** | RW Johnson/Pew Charitable Trusts | $350,000 | Urban | No | Advisory |

This grant essentially provided start-up funds for the MSM Master of Public Health program, which continues to thrive. The MPH program had, and has, an Advisory Committee consisting of academicians, public health professionals, and health advocates.

Dates	Program	Funding source	Amount	Setting		Type
1993–99	Interdisciplinary Training for Health Care for Rural Areas	Health Resources and Services Administration	$1,059,347	Rural	No	Governance

This was a federally funded program carried out through one of the AHEC centers. It offered a summer experience for students of medicine, nursing, and other health professions in rural health centers. The AHEC Program Office Advisory Committee served as an advisory committee, and the Board of Directors of the AHEC Center located in Dublin, GA, served in a governance capacity.

| 1997–2003 | Hamilton Fish Institute of School and Community Violence | US Department of Justice (George Washington University Contract) | $660,000 | Urban | Yes | Advisory |

A citizens' coalition board was organized to address issues of violence in metro Atlanta. The coalition membership included pastors, the Boys and Girls Club of Atlanta, the Metro Atlanta Violence Prevention partnership (another coalition), the Martin Luther King Jr. Center for Social Change, and community residents. A research project was implemented on violence prevention using an evidence-based intervention delivered by educators, clergy, law enforcement officials, and others concerned about youth violence.

| 1997–2000 | Partnerships for Health Professions Education | Health Resources and Services Administration | $1,518,224 | Urban | Yes | Advisory |

A K–16 pipeline program that established initiatives at public schools and HBCUs to encourage and recruit students to pursue health professions careers. It had an advisory committee that consisted of educators from participating public schools and HBCUs.

| 1997–2000 | Breast Health Information & Evaluation (BRIE) | Department of Defense | $583,153 | Rural | No | Advisory |

A research project to test several videotaped dramatizations as mammography motivators. The research participants were African American women in rural Georgia. The project had an advisory committee composed primarily of academics and communication professionals.

| 1998–2024 | Prevention Research Center | Centers for Disease Control and Prevention (CDC) | $18,400,000 | Urban | Yes | Governance |

The MSM PRC is one of a network of academic research centers funded by CDC to achieve local and national health objectives focused on gaining knowledge about the best methodologies for solving the nation's obstinate health problems. The theme of the MSM PRC is Risk Reduction and Early Detection in African American and Other Minority Communities: Coalition for Prevention Research. The mission is to advance scientific knowledge in the field of prevention in African American and other minority communities and to disseminate new information and strategies of prevention. The research focus of MSM PRC includes reduction of HIV risk behavior, cancer prevention, youth violence prevention and reduction, adolescent health promotion, men's health promotion, environmental health and cardiovascular disease prevention. It focuses on reducing health disparities in African American and other minority communities and models ethical approaches to conducting research (community-based participatory research) in these communities. Its Community Coalition Board exercises a governance function. MSM PRC is governed by a Community Coalition Board (CCB), which was established in 1999. It operates under bylaws that were created shortly after the FRC was established. The CCB serves as a policy-making board for the PRC—not an "advisory board." The board is composed of a representative from each of our partners, categorized as academic institutions, agencies, and community neighborhoods. Each of the appointees represents their neighborhood organizations, and community neighborhoods constitute the majority of board membership. The role of the CCB is to (a) set policy and oversee the operations of the center, (b) identify priorities and approve projects, (c) provide information on center activities to the organizations and agencies represented on the board, and (d) develop a strategic plan by which the center may achieve its long-term objectives. The community representatives are always in the majority, and the chair of the board is always a neighborhood representative.

(continued)

Table 4.1 (continued)

Year(s)	Title	Agency	Amount	Urban/rural	Consumer-dominated coalition	Structure governance or advisory
2001–6	**Research on Community Cancer Control**	Centers for Disease Control	$1,291,011	Urban	Yes (2 coalitions)	Governance & Advisory

This was a research grant to test interventions to promote colorectal cancer screening in African Americans. The interventions were developed by a community coalition that consisted of cancer advocates, cancer survivors, and health professionals, acting in an advisory capacity, but the project was carried out by the Prevention Research Center, whose Community Coalition Board is a governing board.

Year(s)	Title	Agency	Amount	Urban/rural	Consumer-dominated coalition	Structure governance or advisory
2006–10	**Community Networks Program**	National Cancer Institute	$6,000,000	Urban	Yes	Governance

Community Networks Program (National Black Leadership Initiative on Cancer, NBLIC): This was a national program, funded by NCI, and headquartered at MSM. Community coalitions were organized in multiple cities across the United States. Each coalition consisted of cancer survivors, cancer advocates, and health professionals, and each coalition carried out its own program of cancer prevention. They could be viewed as performing a self-governance function.

Year(s)	Title	Agency	Amount	Urban/rural	Consumer-dominated coalition	Structure governance or advisory
2007–22	**Clinical and Translational Science Award (CTSA)—Community Engagement Program**	National Center for Resources Research; National Center for Advancing Translational Science	$3,500,000	Urban and Rural	Yes	Governance

The Community Engagement Program of the Georgia CTSA maintains a steering board. This governing body ensures that research findings and related innovations are conducted ethically. It promotes their translation into community practice. The steering board includes a community majority representation, and the board's bylaws require that the chair is a community representative. The board supports community-university research partnerships, obtains community input into university research, and increases health research in community settings that is responsive to the health needs of the community. It connects existing academic community research programs from MSM, Emory University, Georgia Institute of Technology, and the University of Georgia. It strives to transform research from a scientist-subject interaction to an equitable partnership and trains investigators in principles of community-based participatory research. It builds community capacity to conduct collaborative research projects to address critical public health needs.

Year(s)	Title	Agency	Amount	Urban/rural	Consumer-dominated coalition	Structure governance or advisory
2007–22	**Comprehensive Cancer Center / Minority-Serving Institution Partnership**	National Cancer Institute	$1,379,760	Urban and rural	No	Advisory

This project promotes collaboration in cancer research and training among its three partners: University of Alabama at Birmingham Comprehensive Cancer Center, Tuskegee University, and MSM. It has both an Internal Advisory Committee—composed of faculty and staff from the three partners—and an External Advisory Committee, composed of cancer research experts from throughout the United States. The Internal Advisory Committee includes among its members staff that serve the community engagement component of the program, but there is no actual community representation on either committee. Both committees are advisory.

| 2007–12 | **Racial and Ethnic Approaches to Community Health across the U.S. (REACH)** | Centers for Disease Control | $4,250,000 | Urban and Rural | Yes | Governing |

The Southeastern US Collaborative Center of Excellence in the Elimination of Health Disparities (SUCCEED) was created as a response to disproportionately higher breast and cervical cancer incidence and mortality rates among African American women. Its goal was to reduce and eliminate disparities in late-stage diagnosis of breast and cervical cancer between African American and European American women. SUCCEED comprised a lead institution, MSM, and collaborators including Emory University, the Fulton County (GA) Department of Health and Wellness, the Medical University of South Carolina, and the University of North Carolina at Chapel Hill (Primary Partners). SUCCEED promoted breast and cervical cancer screening among medically underserved African American women in Georgia, North Carolina, and South Carolina. The MSM PRC Community Coalition Board served as the governing board for this collaborative.

| 2009–11 | **Multidisciplinary Approach Building Youth: A Prevention and Intervention Program [1]** | Department of Justice, Office of Justice Programs, Office of Juvenile Justice and Delinquency Prevention | $1,000,000 | Urban and Rural | No | Advisory |

Multidisciplinary Approach Building Youth: A Prevention and Intervention Program: An 18-month grant to develop a community-level prevention and intervention collaborative to decrease juvenile delinquency in five Georgia counties (urban and rural). Worked with diverse community organizations and institutions to create an infrastructure to serve the needs of at-risk youth and families to build resiliency among youth. Each interdisciplinary collaborative created a family-centered plan to address needs of program participants. Communication and collaboration improved among participating agencies (e.g., education, social services, mental health, public health, faith institutions, and youth service agencies), and at-risk behavior decreased among program participants. [1] An advisory board of representatives from education, social services, and public and mental health developed action plans.

| 2012–18 | **Reducing Health Disparities in Vulnerable African American Families and Communities** | National Institutes on Minority Health and Health Disparities | $4,484,235 | Urban | No | Advisory |

This project established a Center of Excellence in Health Disparities that focused its efforts on vulnerable African American families and communities. Research projects were implemented in the areas of (1) incarcerated populations and reentry, (2) parent education, and (3) the effects of secondhand smoke on children. Each project had a faculty investigator and was overseen and reviewed by a 20-member community- and consumer-dominated coalition under the auspices of the MSM PRC. The PRC served as a community-level IRB for the research projects. Other activities involved monthly didactic health seminars for community and students and four pilot study projects by junior faculty.

| 2014–16 | **Georgia Strategic Alcohol Prevention Project [2]** | Georgia Department of Behavioral Health and Developmental Disabilities | $200,000 | Rural | Yes | Governance |

This was a multiyear project to address underage and binge drinking among young people ages 18–26 in three rural middle Georgia counties. It created a multicounty collaborative that developed a data-driven strategic plan to address underage and heavy/binge drinking in the target area. It improved the involvement of local law enforcement in preventing underage and binge drinking. In one county, in partnership with the Chamber of Commerce, decreased signage and promotion of alcohol in retail establishments in the three-county area was required for renewal of liquor licenses. [2] A Community Prevention Alcohol Work Group conducted a community assessment and developed a strategic plan to address underage drinking.

(continued)

Table 4.1 (continued)

Year(s)	Title	Agency	Amount	Urban/rural	Consumer-dominated coalition	Structure governance or advisory
2015–19	**MSM—Teenage Pregnancy Prevention Initiative**	Federal Office of Adolescent Health	$1,249,999	Urban and Rural	Yes	Advisory

This project created the Morehouse School of Medicine—Teenage Pregnancy Prevention Initiative (MSM-TPPI). This was a five-year grant to address teenage pregnancy in five diverse Georgia counties, rural and metropolitan. The goal was to provide abstinence-only and comprehensive sex education to over 1,000 middle and high school students. Each program created a community advisory board (CAB) and youth leadership team (YLT) to promote the implementation and sustainability of the program. The active involvement of the CABs increased collaboration among key community stakeholders to sustain prevention activities. Because of the support and involvement of the CABs, the project exceeded the target reach and generated community support for program sustainability after federal funding. Interim data indicate an annual decrease in teenage pregnancies and sexually transmitted diseases in the target communities.

Year(s)	Title	Agency	Amount	Urban/rural	Consumer-dominated coalition	Structure governance or advisory
2013–16	**Using Quality Parenting (UQP) to Address Health Inequities**	National Institutes on Minority Health and Health Disparities	$712,707	Urban	Yes	Governance

The UQP was developed through a partnership between the Satcher Health Leadership Institute (SHLI) and neighborhood residents and organizations in City of Atlanta Neighborhood Planning Units (NPUs) L, T, V, X, Y, and Z. It was built on the lessons learned from the SHLI Smart and Secure Children Program and was guided by the MSM PRC Community Coalition Board model and CBPR approaches. First, a community health needs assessment took place. The survey was designed to find out the child health priorities of adults. Focus groups and community meetings then took place in which residents discussed child health viewpoints and priorities. This information was then used to pilot the UQP intervention serving parents of children ages 6–14 with the overarching aim to promote quality parenting to address community-identified health inequities in early and middle childhood. Planning, implementation, evaluation, and dissemination phases of this grant were led by a community-majority board composed of community leaders. The board was developed and adapted from the MSM PRC research governance model.

Year(s)	Title	Agency	Amount	Urban/rural	Consumer-dominated coalition	Structure governance or advisory
2014–?	**Racial and Ethnic Approaches to Community Health**	Centers for Disease Control and Prevention	$3,680,000	Urban	Yes	Advisory

This comprehensive implementation grant partnered the MSM PRC with the Satcher Health Leadership Institute, Georgia State University, and the National Center for Primary Care. It employed an evidence-based and culturally tailored model that bridges community and clinical connections and tailored policy, systems, and environmental change advised by the MSM PRC Community Coalition Board and other partner communities. Strategies will be designed to improve access to quality health care and reduce risk factors for diabetes and cardiovascular disease among vulnerable adult African Americans. MSM REACH HI will accomplish this through a community-based participatory approach that connects residents to care through community health workers, enlists the clinical leadership of federally qualified health centers, improves behavioral health and chronic disease management, engages community leaders, and improves health outcomes.

1998–2009	**Community Voices**	Kellogg Foundation	$70,000,000	Rural and Urban	Yes	Advisory

Community Voices had its coordinating center housed at MSM. The program involved eight communities (originally 13) across the United States and was dedicated to improving access to health services for underserved populations including low-income groups, racial and ethnic minorities, under- and uninsured immigrants, and other vulnerable populations such as ex-offenders, the incarcerated, and the homeless. The eight sites coordinated by MSM included projects in California, Maryland, Michigan, New York, Florida, North Carolina, New Mexico, and Colorado. All of these implementation sites employed aspects of the Morehouse Model and involved local coalition as part of their change strategy.

2012–17	**Efficacy to Effectiveness Transition of an Educational Program to Increase Colorectal Cancer Screening**	National Cancer Institute	$2,284.95	Urban	Yes	Governance

This was a follow-up project to the Community Cancer Control project. It was a dissemination and implementation research project that utilized the NBLIC community coalitions. Each coalition was invited to participate by implementing, under a variety of conditions, the colorectal cancer screening intervention identified in the Community Cancer Control project. The intervention was named EPICS (Educational Program to Increase Colorectal Cancer Screening). Again, the coalitions were performing a governance (as opposed to advisory) function.

1992–97	**Community Partnerships for Health Professions Education**	Kellogg Foundation	$5,000,000	Urban	Yes	Governance

The goal of this project was to move a major portion of the medical school curriculum into the community, in partnership with several other health professions education programs. This was accomplished by creating a new not-for-profit corporation, the Southeastern Primary Care Consortium, which resembled an AHEC center (in fact, it later assumed the functions of the Atlanta AHEC and became the SPCC/Atlanta AHEC). As a nonprofit corporation it has a board of directors that is a community coalition consisting of health professionals, academicians, and consumers. The Board of Directors performs a governance function. The current community health course (chap. 2) was created as part of this project.

2018–19	**Annie E. Casey Foundation Community Safety Pilot Evaluation**	Annie E. Casey Foundation	$159, 359	Urban	Yes	Advisory

The MSM PRC Evaluation and Institutional Assessment (EIA) Unit engaged in strategic, participatory formative evaluation activities to provide the Annie E. Casey Foundation (AECF) and its partners with data to contribute to continuous improvement efforts, inform potential future implementation of a Community Safety Initiative, and establish baseline data on frequency of acts of crime, particularly gun violence, and residents' overall well-being and perception of safety. A community-based participatory evaluation approach was employed through engagement of multilevel stakeholders who were engaged to inform approaches designed to develop a neighborhood-led, evidence-based, and culturally relevant pilot implementation plan. The MSM PRC EIA Unit collaborated with AECF, a resident advisory committee (RAC) established and composed of six NPU-V community residents for a six-month planning phase. During its second phase, a community-based participatory evaluation approach was employed through engagement of multilevel stakeholders to inform approaches designed to develop and implement a neighborhood-led, evidence-based, and culturally relevant CSP logic model and developmental evaluation. The developmental evaluation will provide AECF and its partners with data to develop and refine the design and processes used in the CSP project, explore the barriers and facilitators to implementation of the project, and explore the barriers and facilitators to stakeholder engagement in the project. Results will inform future outcome and impact evaluation plans and implementation.

(continued)

Table 4.1 (continued)

Year(s)	Title	Agency	Amount	Urban/ rural	Consumer-dominated coalition	Structure governance or advisory
2018–23	**Center for Translational Research in Health Disparities (U54)**	National Institute for Minority Health and Health Disparities	$21,478,330	Urban	Yes	Governance

This five-year project is designed to implement a cohesive multidisciplinary translational team using innovative procedures of bringing combined, integrated, interdisciplinary expertise to bear on health disparities in and with local communities as mentees in women's health research dealing with basic science and behavioral science studies, directed by three faculty investigators. The community coalition board under the auspices of the MSM PRC serves as the CE entity for interfacing with the research projects. The PRC has a review committee that serves as the community IRB and has the responsibility of reviewing the faculty-led research projects for scientific integrity and human subject ethics. In community topical seminars, workshops and training events are planned for implementation during the coming year.

The 32 grants noted in table 4.1 capture the lion's share of the funded projects where CE and community coalition building were part of the implementation goals. While this list is not exhaustive, it highlights the sustained and ongoing involvement of MSM with community coalition building dating back to the institution's early beginnings. The institution has had six presidents since its inception, and all of them have shown a strong commitment to primary care and involving consumers and health and human service agencies in the work of the institution. This type of consistent leadership from the top has enabled MSM's brand to be well established among medical schools in America; that brand can best be characterized as a commitment to health equity, social justice, and a consistency of social mission. The brand has been manifested through effective teaching, research, and service to communities throughout Georgia and the Southeast region, and in some cases nationally.

How Did MSM Become Uniquely Established for This CE Brand?

It is important to note that MSM faculty are not "helicopter researchers," who fly into communities, collect data, and abscond to publish papers. No, the majority of the faculty are passionately committed to working collaboratively with communities in a participatory manner. As reported in the *Annals of Internal Medicine* in 2010,[3] MSM was the leading medical school in the nation in the area of social mission among the 140 US osteopathic and allopathic medical schools. Data were analyzed to rank physicians' alma maters in three dimensions: production of primary care physicians, underrepresented minority graduates, and graduates practicing in medically underserved areas.

This MSM recognition reemphasizes the importance of the MSM mission at a critical time in which the nation needs to reform its health system with a strong focus on primary care. MSM is at the epicenter of the movement. This position builds on our long-standing reputation of training the doctors America needs most. Moreover, it draws national attention to our unique position as the nation seeks new approaches and new alternatives to addressing the vexing challenges of affordable health and health care, expanding the number of primary care physicians and critical specialists working in underserved communities, increasing the racial and ethnic diversity in the health professions, eliminating racial and geographic ethnic health inequities, and reducing preventable deaths and promoting healthier lifestyles.

In January 2011, the Carnegie Foundation for the Advancement of Teaching awarded its CE recognition to MSM. "The Carnegie Classification for Community Engagement is like a Good Housekeeping Seal of Approval indicating that the medical school and the communities are partners," according to Donna Gessell from Carnegie. Carnegie specifically defines engagement as collaboration between a university and its region for the mutually beneficial exchange of knowledge and resources. In April 2011, the MSM Prevention Research Center was recognized by the Centers for Disease Control and Prevention as having a model approach to community-based participatory research.

MSM was founded by visionaries with a passionate commitment to "serve the underserved." Over its 40-year history, MSM established an intimate relationship and bond of trust with numerous minority communities. MSM has achieved national stature based on its trailblazing focus on community outreach and primary care delivery programs to high health disparity neighborhoods. It is noted that minority-serving academic health centers that have earned the trust of underserved communities are poised to play a pivotal role in providing scientific and human service leadership that advances the health status of populations of color. In our view, full institutional commitment to diversity is measured by diversity among, within, and across faculty ranks. The absence of a diversified faculty is a failure of the diversity litmus test, which must be administered to advance health disparity research.[2]

As MSM and especially the Department of Community Health and Preventive Medicine seek to advance the discipline of prevention science, we must realize the need for continuous evaluation of the Morehouse Model for CE. There are at least four areas where new and expanded work is needed to advance CE efforts at MSM, and indeed across the nation. Those areas are voter rights and voter registration, job creation, participatory budgeting (PB), and CE coalitions as a tool for social justice. These areas will be discussed in the following sections.

Voter Rights and Registration

A 2012 study by the Pew Charitable Trusts estimated that 24 percent of the voting-eligible population in the United States was not registered to vote.[4] This represents about 51 million citizens. As we move forward with advancing the Morehouse Model, including a voter registration component is essential to maximizing CE. Thus, voter rights and registration will be offered as an ongoing training and technical assistance area for coalitions and consumer constituents. This inclusion is tantamount for effective CE, given the recent voter suppression claims here in Georgia with the 2018 governor's race and elsewhere. It has been noted that numerous states have a history of creating barriers to voter registration through a variety of fees, literacy or comprehension tests, and record-keeping practices that discriminate against racial and ethnic minorities. Despite the passage of the Voting Rights Act of 1963, some states continue to develop new practices that discriminate against certain populations. By August 2016, federal rulings in five cases had overturned all or parts of voter registration or voter ID laws in Ohio, Texas, North Carolina, Wisconsin, and North Dakota that were found to place a burden on minorities and other groups.[5, 6]

While voters traditionally had to register at government offices by a certain period before an election, in the mid-1990s the federal government made efforts to simplify registration procedures to improve access and increase turnout. The National Voter Registration Act of 1993 (also known as the "Motor Voter Act") required state governments to either provide uniform opt-in registration services through drivers' license registration centers, disability centers, schools, libraries, and mail-in registration or allow voter registration on Election Day, where voters can register at polling places immediately prior to voting. On January 1, 2016, Oregon became the first state to adopt a fully automatic voter registration system as part of the process of issuing driver licenses and ID cards. By April 2016 three more states—California, West

Virginia, and Vermont—had followed suit, and in May 2016 Connecticut implemented it administratively rather than by legislation, bringing the number of states with automatic voter registration to five.[7-10]

Voter rights and registration in the Black community and especially in the "Bible Belt" southern states have been marked by confrontation, protest, and litigation. You may be familiar with the protest march from Selma to Montgomery, Alabama—which became labeled as "Bloody Sunday." During this March 7, 1965, march of 600 voting rights activists, led by John Lewis of the Student Nonviolent Coordinating Committee and Hosea Williams of the Southern Christian Leadership Council, marchers were brutally attacked by Alabama state troopers wearing gas masks, along with local police and a posse on horseback. Worldwide attention to the Selma marches finally forced Congress to pass legislation that would guarantee voting rights for all Americans. President Lyndon B. Johnson signed the Voting Rights Act into law on August 6, 1965. This is only part of the long history and legacy of fighting for voting rights in the United States. This was the beginning of the end to the "jelly bean test"—where the voter registrar would ask minority voters to guess the number of jelly beans in a jar.

So here we are in 2020, and the more things change, the more they stay the same, as evidenced by voter suppression tactics employed by unscrupulous and mean-spirited election officials. A more recent case of election fraud was well documented during the 2018 Ninth Congressional race in North Carolina. In a close race a political operative had encouraged voters to request absentee ballots, which he collected and allegedly turned in to election officials. Such behavior is illegal in North Carolina and was deemed as a form of ballot tampering. The disputed close race in this district and the observation of election fraud, not fraud by voters, resulted in the state election board ordering a new election more than three months after the November 6, 2018, election.[11]

While we are more than 50 years removed from the confrontation on the Edmund Pettus Bridge on "Bloody Sunday," the tactics have grown to be more sophisticated and systematic. We now have "exact match" practices by voter registrars, where an omitted hyphen in one's name can be the difference between being allowed to vote and not being allowed to vote. Voting is the highest level of civil responsibility and indeed a segue to citizen participation and CE. For these reasons, and given the history of voter suppression, voter registration has evolved as a critical and new component of the Morehouse Model. Thus, voter registration activities will be incorporated as a viable component of new CE efforts.

Participatory Budgeting

As we continue to advance new knowledge in CE methods, Morehouse is eager to embrace the PB movement, now being implemented by a select few municipalities across the country. We will advocate for PB with local counties and cities throughout Georgia and the southern states. We will also employ PB with mini-grants to community groups in the Atlanta area. So, what exactly is PB? PB is a democratic process of CE in which community residents determine how to spend part of a public budget. It gives real power over real public dollars. This is a rather new approach to citizen involvement in municipal decision-making about how to allocate tax dollars. PB is manifested with an annual cycle of engagement that is integrated into a local government's regular budgeting process and includes the following five phases over the course of a fiscal year:

1. *Design the process.*—This begins with a steering committee that represents the community. This steering committee creates the rules for an engagement plan.
2. *Brainstorming of ideas.*—Through meetings and online tools, residents share and discuss ideas for development projects.
3. *Develop proposals.*—Volunteer "budget delegates" develop the ideas into feasible proposals.
4. *Vote.*—Residents vote on the proposals that most serve the community needs.
5. *Fund winning projects.*—The local government funds and implements the winning ideas.[11, 12]

The first full PB process was birthed in Porto Alegra, Brazil.[12, 13] Unsurprisingly, this was the birth country of Paulo Freire, the world-renowned Brazilian educator, philosopher, and internationally recognized guru of community organizing. He authored *Pedagogy of the Oppressed* in 1970.[13, 14] In 1969, after his work in educating and organizing the disenfranchised was internationally recognized, he was offered a visiting professorship at Harvard University. He was known as a Christian Socialist, and following his year at Harvard he went to work in Geneva for the World Council of Churches, where he became an education advisor for several countries in Africa. In 1988, he was appointed secretary of education for Brazil.

In the Porto Alegra PB model the structure of the scheme gives subjurisdictions (neighborhoods) authority over the larger political jurisdictions (the city) of which they are a part. Neighborhood budget committees had the authority to determine the citywide budget, not just the allocation of resources for their particular neighborhood. Thus, there was a need for mediating institutions to facilitate the aggregation of budget preferences as expressed by subjurisdictions.

According to the World Bank Group, certain factors are needed for PB to be adopted, such as "strong mayoral support, a civil society willing and able to contribute to ongoing policy debates, a generally supportive political environment that insulates participatory budgeting from legislators' attacks, and financial resources to fund the projects selected by citizens." In addition, there are generally two approaches through which PB formulates: top-down and bottom-up.[14, 15] The adoption of PB has been required by the federal government in Peru, while there are cases in which local governments initiated PB independent from the national agenda, such as Porto Alegre. With the bottom-up approach, nongovernmental organizations (NGOs) and local organizations have played a crucial role in mobilizing and informing the community members.

As of July 2019, PB has been implemented in 148 sites in the United States, and citizens have directly decided how to spend $306 million and empowered more than 600,000 citizens according to the national PB organization.[11, 12, 15]

The impacts of this movement include increased civic engagement; stronger and more collaborative relationships between residents, government, and community-based organizations; more inclusive political

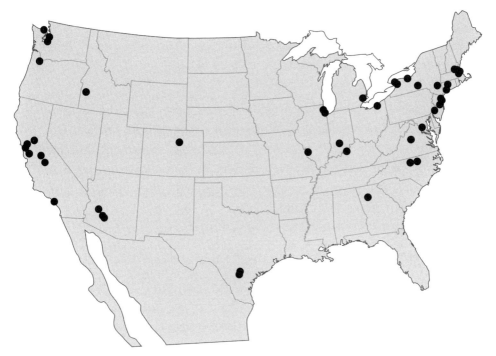

Map of participatory budgeting sites in the United States as of 2019

participation (especially by historically marginalized communities); new community leaders; and more equitable and effective public spending. The PB process is being implemented in large cities and small towns across the United States, such as New York City, Oakland, Phoenix, Boston, Seattle, Greensboro, and Minneapolis. Atlanta is a new city coming online with PB. Several of the beta sites for PB will be described within this chapter as case study presentations. According to the PB national project, PB is occurring in over 3,000 cities around the world.[11,][12] PB has been recognized as a best practice for CE by the following:

- The US Conference of Mayors
- National League of Cities
- US Department of Housing and Urban Development
- The Obama White House
- Harvard University—Ash Center for Democratic Governance and Innovation

- 10 Resilient Cities
- The Movement for Black Lives
- The Aspen Institute
- Policy Link

The National PB project provides direct support and technical assistance on PB to help local governments improve their PB process. This includes providing trainings, tools, and coaching to assist with the high-impact CE process to advance equity in citizen decision-making over public dollars. This is truly a process of giving citizens a "seat at the table," thus taking them "off the menu."

How Much Money Is Enough to Do PB?

According to the PB Project officials in Brooklyn, New York, PB can be implicated with varying amounts of fiscal resources. They suggest that most PB processes use between 1 and 15 percent of the local city's budget. For larger municipalities they suggest $1 million per 100,000 residents, so that the invitation to participate is compelling. Though PB can be done with any amount of money, the more funds that are available, the more potential impact the process will have on CE and citizen buy-in. The PB Project officials indicate that in some places PB has been written into law through a charter modification. Such a change is useful for the long-term visibility of the process and public transparency. However, since the vast majority of PB processes use discretionary funds, there is no need for legislation to begin the process, according to the PB Project officials. They indicate that all it takes to start the process is the political will and commitment of decision-makers. Here, there is no need to change who holds budgetary authority.[11, 12]

Examples of PB

In December 2018, Atlanta city council member Amir Farokhi introduced legislation that would amend the city charter to fund PB in Atlanta. With PB programs, Farokhi says, "residents will propose capital projects for their communities, create a ballot of the best ideas, and vote on projects to implement free of local government interference." He goes on to indicate that PB programs have been successfully implemented in the United States and globally, from Seattle and Chicago to Paris and Madrid. Farokhi hopes to get funding for his pilot as part of the fiscal year 2020 budget, which was reviewed for approval in June 2019.[15, 16]

Chicago PB

PB Chicago is a broad coalition of aldermen, city agencies, CBOs, and residents working to implement and expand PB processes and direct democracy throughout Chicago. Since 2012, the Great Cities Institute has been the lead university partner on PB Chicago, responsible for stewarding the initiative, as well as providing overall project management, training, and technical assistance on CE and evaluation. In 2009, residents of Chicago's Forty-Ninth Ward held the first PB vote in the United States, led by Alderman Joe Moore. In 2012, the third year of PB voting in Chicago, PB Chicago was formed to help support, implement, and expand PB processes across the city. Since then, Chicago residents in participating aldermanic wards have voted on how to spend the $1 million in "menu money" for infrastructure improvements that the city council allocates to each ward. PB Chicago has successfully implemented six voting cycles across the city (and currently is in the seventh cycle), engaging more than 26,000 residents in 12 wards in directly deciding how to spend approximately $31 million on over 160 community projects. With the support of the Great Cities Institute and its coalition of PB supporters around the city, in recent years PB Chicago has supported and expanded "menu money" votes around aldermanic infrastructure funds. PB Chicago also led the country's first PB process with tax increment financing money in the United States, a vote that was held in Chicago's West Humboldt Park community. And in 2017, PB Chicago began working with Chicago Public Schools to pilot a PB-based CE program for high schoolers. In 2018, PB Chicago partnered with Our City Our Voice to continue providing technical assistance and support to PB processes across the city. Since that time, Chicago residents have fixed streets and sidewalks, improved parks, built out biking and transit infrastructure, updated libraries and schools, and more.[16, 17]

New York City PB

According to recent reports from the Participatory Budgeting Organization, for the seventh year in a row New Yorkers have participated in the PB process of deciding part of the city budget. In 2018 more than 99,250 residents age 11 and older participated in the largest civic engagement program in the United States by deciding how to spend $36.5 million across New York City. Through PB they developed hundreds of spending proposals and funded 124 community improvement projects for schools, parks, libraries, public housing, streets, and other public spaces. The impacts of PB are even greater over time. Since 2012, New Yorkers have decided how to spend $210 million on 706 projects.[11, 12]

The PB organization also reported that they have launched a new data tool for monitoring the implementation of projects, once funded. The tool was developed in response to the lack of a comprehensive city-wide view and measure of PB-funded projects. The new data tool (myPB) monitors status and outcomes. The tool is being pilot tested in New York City and will be available to other municipalities engaging PB. The link for the myPB data tool is http://mypb.community.

Community Development Block Grants

Some urban planners suggest that PB has taken the Community Development Block Grant (CDBG) program to a higher level. CDBG is a federal program under the auspices of the US Department of Housing and Urban Development.[11, 12] The intent of CDBG was to fund local community development activities such as affordable housing, anti-poverty programs, and infrastructure development. This program was created in 1974 by President Gerald Ford through the Housing and Community Development Act of 1974 and took effect in January 1975. The idea was to move away from categorical grants made for specific purposes and to give local and state governments and their subgrantees more authority and decision-making on how to allocate dollars for local needs. The major pitfall of the CDBG program was the lack of citizen involvement, while the state and local macroagency personnel maintained decision-making authority over how these funds were to be spent. PB uses an intentional strategy for involving local residents in the decision-making processes.

Job Creation for CE

Although many job opportunities have been created through the funded grants implemented while applying the Morehouse Model, job creation has emerged as an institutionalized element of the model. One could effectively argue that job creation as it relates to community development has been a missing link. When you consider the "town and gown" relationship between MSM and the many community coalitions with which we have collaborated, it would be prudent for the medical school to provide intentional leadership for a job creation/job development component as part of the Morehouse Model.

Job creation/job development has many facets, including education, training, and placement. Community organizers meeting residents at the grassroots level invariably encounter citizens in need of employment. Hence, advocating for job creation, development, and placement is definitely a win-win activity. It is a win-win for the community, the academic partner, and the coalition.

It is not uncommon in urban inner-city areas to encounter ex-offenders who are seeking to rejuvenate their lives but are confronted with barriers due to a criminal record. Counseling, coaching, and advocating for this population are important community development and CE tasks, essential for building trust and restoring the dignity of ex-offenders seeking to rebuild their lives. Having knowledge about companies that are friendly to hiring ex-offenders is a useful resource for all community coalitions. According to a recent count, there are 275 national companies that hire ex-offenders.[17, 18] Among these companies were:

- Alamo Rent a Car
- Allstate Insurance
- Amazon
- American Airlines
- Budget Rent a Car
- Chase Bank
- The Coca Cola Company
- Comcast
- Domino's Pizza
- Google
- Greyhound
- Hilton Hotels
- Apple Inc.
- AT&T
- Avis Rent a Car
- Bed, Bath, and Beyond
- Holiday Inn
- Home Depot
- Lowe's
- McDonald's
- Starbucks
- Uber
- Wal-Mart

Community Health Workers and Job Creation

Within the CE space university faculty who advocate for CBPR have embraced the notion that lay personnel are an essential part of outreach to local residents. Across the United States and at the international level indigenous citizens have been trained to recruit and transmit health education and prevention information to local residents. The concept is not new and has been used around the world in Peace Corps projects. Workers within this emerging job classification have been called community health workers, patient navigators, and promotores. They function as a trusted link between macroagencies and local residents. Their mission is to connect local residents to health and human services available at the macroagency level. For example, they might typically work with a family to acquire health insurance benefits and assist them with completing an application for the Affordable Care Act benefits or health benefit programs offered by a local or state agency, or they might serve as organizers and conveners of a coalition to acquire categorical health benefits, such as mental health, housing, or substance abuse assistance. The idea is that the CHW is savvy and serves as a "code switcher" for advocating for the client with health and human service providers.

The Morehouse Model implementers have stimulated the growth of CHW throughout many of its projects, thus helping to stimulate a new career for these lay citizens. Many macro-organizations and NGOs recruit and hire staff with experience as CHWs. At MSM a CHW certification program has been launched for the state of Georgia. This topic is discussed in greater detail in chapter 6.

Coalition CE as a Tool for Social Justice

Coalitions are not a new concept but have gained increased recognition as a social change methodology. A case in point are the efforts of Colin Kaepernick, a former quarterback for the San Francisco 49ers. Since August 2016, following his example, some American athletes have protested against police brutality and racism by kneeling during the playing of the US national anthem. The protests began in the National Football League (NFL) after Kaepernick sat and later knelt during the anthem, before one of his team's preseason games in 2016. Throughout the following seasons, members of various NFL and other sports teams have engaged in coalition-like behavior in similar silent protests. On September 24, 2017, the NFL protest became more widespread, when over 200 players sat or knelt in response to President Donald Trump calling for owners to "fire" the protesting players.[18, 19]

Criminal justice reform is currently a top issue that the NFL players have been supporting in their protests. Kaepernick was initially moved to protest by the deaths of African Americans at the hands of police or while in police custody. These deaths gained prominence through the media and the Black Lives Matter movement in the years immediately preceding the protest. During a postgame interview on August 26, 2016, Kaepernick stated, "I am not going to stand up to show pride in a flag for a country that oppresses Black people and people of color. To me, this is bigger than football and it would be selfish on my part to look the other way. There are bodies in the street and people getting paid leave and getting away with murder," adding that he would continue to protest during the anthem until he feels like "[the US flag] represents what it is supposed to represent." After that interview, Kaepernick pledged to donate the first $1 million of his $11.9 million salary from the 2016–17 season to different organizations that assist communities in need. Several days later the San Francisco 49ers matched Kaepernick by pledging $1 million to two organizations addressing racial and social inequality. Kaepernick followed through and has made donations to Meals on Wheels, United We Dream, and Black Veterans for Social Justice, among many others. The NFL Players Association named Kaepernick the Week One Community MVP in September 2017 for his charity work related to protest.[19, 20]

This is a story and a case study that most people know and have heard about. The several and varying spins and interpretations that have been attributed to Kaepernick's kneeling are well known. Many call it unpatriotic, in spite of his efforts to clarify that his behavior was not about disrespecting the flag or veterans. We mention the Kaepernick case to illustrate the point that a coalition can be ignited by a compelling issue of concern to the masses. The Kaepernick protest has morphed into a national CE movement involving Nike and the NFL launching its Players Coalition social justice program, "Inspire Change"; collaborations with Big Brothers Big Sisters of America; and Operation HOPE, which will establish a digital learning curriculum for African Americans in 175 high schools. In 2018 the NFL donated $8.5 million, plus $2 million for NFL Foundation grants for clubs, former players, and active players. The NFL promises to donate $100 million to charities and organizations that support law enforcement relationships with communities, criminal justice reform, and education reform.[20, 21]

The Women's Movement

The Women's March was a worldwide CE protest that convened January 21, 2017, the day after the inauguration of President Donald Trump. Tensions rose as a result of misogynistic statements made by Donald Trump. It was the largest single-day protest in US history. More than 5 million marchers participated across US cities. Now in its third year, this annual march advocates for legislation and policies regarding human rights and other issues, including women's rights (equal pay for equal work), immigration reform, health care reform, reproductive rights, LGBTQ rights, racial equality, and worker's rights and tolerance.

This coalition of CE marchers included support from Planned Parenthood, AFL-CIO, Amnesty International, the National Organization of Women, MoveOn, Human Rights Watch, Code Pink, Black Girls Rock, the National Association for the Advancement of Colored People (NAACP), the American Indian Movement, Green Peace USA, and the League of Women Voters. More than 100 celebrity supporters endorsed this effort, including the following:

- Ariana Grande
- Cher
- John Legend
- Lupita Nyong'o
- Madonna
- Rihanna
- Chris Rock
- Drew Barrymore
- Julia Roberts
- Zendaya

This coalition demonstrates that the CE is not bound by geography, but rather is a meeting of like-minded people organized to address compelling social justice and equality issues. The Women's March has morphed into the "Me Too" movement, which has exposed hundreds of sexually abusive men. The Women's March has no doubt inspired women to run for elective office at the national, state, and local levels. The 116th Congress has 110 women (81 Democrats and 29 Republicans) holding seats, or 20.6 percent of the 535 members. In the US Senate 23 women (23%) are now seated. The 2020 US presidential race, as of this writing, has observed five women declaring candidacy (Elizabeth Warren, Amy Klobuchar, Tulsi Gabbard, Kirsten Gillibrand, and Kamala Harris). We anticipate even more candidates than the five that have declared. Some prognosticators advance that this is the era for women to coalesce and save America from its downward spiral, but whether they save America or not, it is clear that coalitions will make a difference in legislation and policy issues for many years ahead.

National Coalition on Health Care

The National Coalition on Health Care is a coalition of groups working to achieve comprehensive health system reform. It was founded in 1990 by Dr. Henry Simmons as a nonprofit alliance of more than 80 organizations. The coalition's mission is grounded on five independent principles forming a framework for improving America's health care system. They seek health care coverage for all, cost management, improvement of health care quality and safety, equitable financing, and simplified administration. Some of the member organizations include AARP, AFL-CIO, the American Legacy Foundation, the League of Women Voters, the NAACP, and the National Council of La Raza.

The results of the work of CE and coalitions of all types have undeniably moved the needle for social change and policy initiatives in the United States. Whether they be single-issue-driven coalitions or poly-issue coalitions, they have demonstrated an ability to mobilize masses of people to advocate for social policy positions. While these collaborations have grown exponentially, they are not without flaws that serve to weaken their sustained viability. Hence, many of these groups dissolve and cease to exist owing to internal strife, power struggles, and the lack of strategic planning. More coalitions dissipate and fail than those that are sustained. So, one must ask the question, why do coalitions and CE fail?

Why Do Coalitions and CE Fail?

There are numerous barriers that hurt and cripple coalitions and the CE process. Many of these negative forces can be abated with insight, political astuteness, and diligent planning. Given that those involved with the coalition and CE process are often volunteers, one barrier is volunteer burnout. Sustaining a coalition requires that the organizers maintain an objective of continuing to recruit and orient new coalition members to replace members who will surely resign from the process after a year or two. Some are in for the long haul and stay much longer, but there will undoubtedly be those who withdraw from the coalition or CE process after a relatively short period of time.

"Mission drift" is also a nagging barrier that undermines coalition and CE sustainability. Coalitions, once established, will adopt a mission statement as part of their statement of purpose. Coalition members can be thrown off of the a priori mission by the presentation of new opportunities and resources. This is not to say that an organized coalition cannot have multiple aims. Some coalitions were established with a single focus mission; when that changes by virtue of new opportunities, membership and participation from the entire group may dwindle if branching to new initiatives has not been negotiated with the founding members. Of course, the mission can be changed and evolve by modification and ratification, but these shifts should be addressed forthrightly, with new buy-in from the group, if the group's impetus is to be sustained. Coalitions are also negatively impacted by factions, cliques, and political subgroups within the coalition. This observation will manifest when there becomes an imbalance in decision-making and when one or a fraction of members begin to dominate the discussion on a consistent basis. Rather than operating from a consensus model, the less assertive members begin to feel that their input, ideas, and perspective are not valued. This leads to fracturing and splitting of the collective, and membership participation will wane. Sometimes splintering is more covert yet intentional and manifests as sabotage of the group. This is a more serious behavior and must be confronted with open and heart-to-heart discussion. Sabotage is related to members having a hidden agenda. When hidden agendas are suspected, they need to be respectfully confronted head-on.

Coalitions also fail when consensus decisions are not represented with fidelity. After debating policy or practice issues and following agreement and consensus, the members with opposition ideas must assimilate to the consensus decision. Otherwise, the group will be weakened by backbiting members speaking publicly about a nonconsensus position. Some coalitions collapse when funding resources evaporate. Thus, the presence of money has a "sugar and spice" effect. Some members will participate fully when financial resources are available and then drop off when funding ends. Hence, all coalitions need to engage in a strategic planning process where coalition sustainability is discussed and plans are made to address anticipated financial shortfalls or grant endings. So, the issue to be addressed is, how do we institutionalize, adopt, and maintain some if not all of our programmatic activities? These questions and answers can be addressed with the assistance of external evaluators providing feedback on the strengths and weaknesses of co-alition activities and through use of strategic planning.

Coalitions fail owing to turf issues. Member leadership can often be undermined by feelings that the mission of one's agency is being en-croached upon. This is particularly true when macroagencies become competitive about turf concerns. While coalition failure can be attrib-uted to many of the above-noted issues, coalition sustainability can be achieved with shared leadership, annual recognition, and awards to member volunteers, as well as ongoing coalition training and technical assistance to get ahead of these anticipated barriers and pitfalls.

Summary

Implementing CBPR, coalition development, and CE through the Morehouse Model over the past 40-plus years has afforded MSM fac-ulty an opportunity to provide leadership in attaining health equity for disenfranchised populations. This work began and continues with the primary care mission of the institution and a recognition that many citi-zens are suffering from preventable diseases. While health disparities con-tinue to lead to abysmal outcomes for Black and ethnic minorities, CE has given rise to sustained hope for improved health and an enhanced quality of life despite persistent structural impediments and discrimina-tion. Access to quality health care is inseparable from politics, and CE has evolved into a political process for positive community change.

Achieving healthier communities is punctuated by a thin line between systems blame and personal responsibility. We acknowledge the com-pelling social determinants of health and the systemic impediments while also acknowledging that shifting cultures of personal behavior are also a powerful implement for change. The Morehouse Model for CE and health equity is institutionalized and tantamount to a lifelong institutional legacy of commitments from past presidents to our cur-rent president, Valerie Montgomery Rice, MD. She continues to be bold and provide audacious leadership in "climbing Jacob's Ladder" and brokering, leveraging, and launching new vistas for training socially conscious health professionals.

The many examples of the Morehouse Model and CE noted earlier in this chapter are a good start, but we recognize the need for more intentional work to advance the model. Voter rights and voter registration, job creation strategies, PB, and social justice are value-added components for the Morehouse Model.

References

1. Fiegener, Mark K., and Steven L. Proudfoot. 2013. *Baccalaureate Origins of U.S.-Trained S&E Doctorate Recipients*. Arlington, VA: National Science Foundation, National Center for Science and Engineering Statistics.

2. Treadwell, Henrie M., Ronald L. Braithwaite, Kisha Braithwaite, Desiree Oliver, and Rhonda Holliday. 2009. "Leadership Development for Health Researchers at Historically Black Colleges and Universities." *American Journal of Public Health* 99 (S1): S53–57.

3. Mullan, Fitzhugh, Candice Chen, Stephen Patterson, Gretchen Kolsky, and Michael Spagnola. 2010. "The Social Mission of Medical Education: Ranking the Schools." *Annals of Internal Medicine* 152 (12): 804–11.

4. Pew Charitable Trust. 2012. "Inaccurate, Costly, and Inefficient: Evidence That America's Voter Registration System Needs an Upgrade." Pew Center on the States, February 14, 2012.

5. De Vogue, Ariane. 2016. "Voting Challenges Head toward the Supreme Court: 4 Cases to Watch." CNN, July 19, 2016. https://www.cnn.com/2016/07/19/politics /voting-rights-supreme-court/index.html.

6. Wines, Michael, and Alan Blinder. 2016. "Voter ID Laws Take a Beating in U.S. Courts." *New York Times*, July 29, 2016.

7. Barnes, Robert. 2016. "Federal Judge Blocks N. Dakota's Voter-ID Law, Calling It Unfair to Native Americans." *Washington Post*, August 1, 2016.

8. "Oregon Motor Voter Act FAQ." Oregon Secretary of State. https://sos.oregon .gov/voting/pages/motor-voter-faq.aspx.

9. Brenman Center for Justice. 2016. "The Case for Automatic Voter Registration." Brenman Center for Justice, April 1, 2016. https://www.brennancenter.org/sites /default/files/publications/Case_for_Automatic_Voter_Registration.pdf.

10. "Shumlin Signs into Law Automatic Voter Registration." *Vermont Business Magazine*, April 28, 2016.

11. Berry. D. B. 2019. "Disputed North Carolina House Race: Elections Board Orders New Election." *USA Today*, February 21, 2019.

12. "Participatory Budgeting Project." https://participatorybudgeting.org/.

13. Wampler, Brian. 2007. *Participatory Budgeting in Brazil: Contestation, Cooperation, and Accountability*. University Park: Pennsylvania State University Press.

14. Friere, Paulo. 1970. *Pedagogy of the Oppressed*. New York: Scabury.

15. Shah, Anwar, ed. 2007. *Participatory Budgeting*. Washington, DC: World Bank.

16. "Council Member Amir Farokhi Introduces Bill Proposing 'Participatory Budgeting' Program for Atlanta." *Atlanta Daily World*, December 17, 2018.

17. "Participatory Budgeting." Great Cities Institute, University of Illinois at Chicago. https://greatcities.uic.edu/uic-neighborhoods-initiative/%20participatory -budgeting/.

18. Curtis, Whitney. 2019. "Jobs for Falcons." *New York Times*, January 2019.

19. Associated Press. 2017. "Trump Says NFL Should Fire Players Who Kneel during National Anthem." *Los Angeles Times*, September 22, 2017.

20. Wyche, Stave. 2016. "Colin Kaepernick Explains Why He Sat during National Anthem." NFL.com, August 27, 2016. http://www.nfl.com/news/story /0ap3000000691077/article/colin-kaepernick-explains-why-he-sat-during-national -anthem.

21. Haring, Bruce. 2019. "NFL Launches Its Players Coalition Social Justice Program, 'Inspire Change.'" Deadline.com, January 12, 2019. https://deadline.com /2019/01/nfl-launches-its-players-coalition-social-justice-program-inspire-changes -1202534278/.

FIVE

Engaging Micropolitan and Rural Communities in Health Promotion and Disease Prevention

R URAL AMERICA is less healthy than urban America. Statistics that point to an urban-rural health disparity include a higher rural over-all mortality rate,[1] a higher rural infant mortality rate,[2] and higher rates of individual causes of death, ranging from stroke[3] to suicide.[4] Life expectancy is about two and a half years shorter in rural areas than in metropolitan areas, and this gap is widening.[5] Black-White health disparities are even greater in rural areas than they are in cities.[6]

Often, poor rural health status is attributed to a rural shortage of physicians and other health professionals, the great distances that must be traveled to obtain health care, and a lack of public transportation to facilitate traveling those great distances. There is no doubt that these barriers to obtaining medical care are serious issues, but other matters play important roles as well. According to the National Rural Health Association, "Economic factors, cultural and social differences, educational differences, lack of recognition by legislators and the sheer isolation of living in remote rural areas all conspire to impede rural Americans in their struggle to lead a normal, healthy life."[7] These social determinants lead to risk factors that help explain urban-rural disparities. For instance, smoking, obesity, and lack of leisure-time physical activity are more prevalent in rural than in urban areas.[8]

The United States is in the grip of an opioid overuse epidemic, and this, too, is more prevalent in rural than in urban areas.[9, 10] Hospitalization for prescription opioid overdose is higher in rural than in urban areas,[11] as is overdose more generally.[12] Accidental overdose deaths, like suicides, have come to be known as "deaths of despair" and are associated with unemployment, underemployment, and the effects that these have on one's family and social status. They are more common in rural than in urban areas.[13]

Like nonmedical opioid use, adolescent pregnancy—which is also more common in rural than in urban areas—is likely related to social determinants. Teen birth rates have fallen dramatically since 2007, but in rural areas they remain about 40 percent higher than in urban areas.[14] This is true in Georgia,[15] as well as in the United States generally.

Social determinants, mental health, and related issues are often more effectively addressed by health promotion, broadly defined, than by medical care. However, entities charged with conducting health promotion campaigns in rural communities—primarily public health departments—are chronically underfunded and understaffed. Mental health services in rural areas are scarce. A portion of the health promotion need has been filled by the faith community, particularly (but by no means exclusively) in the African American community. Health promotion campaigns in and through churches have focused on nutrition and physical activity,[16] mental health,[17, 18] smoking cessation,[19] and other matters.

In rural and micropolitan communities, the faith community (i.e., churches, pastors) is an important partner in facilitating community entry, and this is certainly true in Georgia. It does not matter if the pastor is a "circuit pastor," who is not a community resident and lives in another county; his or her support is important in gaining entrance to the minority community. Historically, the church is one of the most important institutions in the African American community because of its dichotomous mission, both spiritual and social. Many educational and social programs started in the Black church and continue to address the needs of vulnerable populations in the community. It is in the Black church that individuals find equality, the educated and the uneducated worshiping and serving together.

Thus, any academic institution wishing to engage a rural African American community for health promotion (or other purposes) would do well to start by engaging the clergy. This is consistent with the Morehouse Model as described in chapter 1. In that model, one starts with a community-based organization (CBO), but in a rural area, there might not be such an organization, or if there is (e.g., social action groups), it might not consider health as one of its primary concerns. A pastor, on the other hand, is generally concerned with the health of his flock, and the church can act as a CBO.

In any case, in a rural community where "everybody knows everybody else," community engagement will need to begin by engaging community leaders. Church leaders will almost always be among them, but others may include public elected officials, health care leaders (e.g., hospital administrator, health department director, medical society president), and prominent businessmen. These individuals will also serve as "key informants" for the process of problem identification, goal setting, and needs assessment—step 2 in the Morehouse Model. Other activities, of course, may include data gathering, surveys, focus groups, and so on, as described in chapter 1. Asset mapping will be important; the wealth of assets to be found in even low-income rural communities is often not recognized. However, it is from these "assets" that partners in coalition building (step 3) will be found. As mentioned, these will include churches, the local hospital, the health department, the medical society or health center, and businesses, as well as the school system, the law enforcement agency, and other public agencies.

These were among the methods employed by the School of Medicine Promotion Resource Center (MSM HPRC), as will be seen from the description of its activities that follow.

The Morehouse School of Medicine Health Promotion Research Center

The MSM HPRC was established in 1988 as a center within the Department of Community Health and Preventive Medicine. Initially funded by the Kaiser Family Foundation in Menlo Park, California, the

HPRC developed a health promotion and disease prevention model for underserved populations, which was the early beginning of the Morehouse Model.

In our work in nonmetropolitan communities (rural and micropolitan), the HPRC applied the following nine basic principles of CE to facilitate our CE efforts for health promotion and disease prevention:[20] (1) be clear about the population/communities to be engaged and the goals of the effort; (2) know the community, including its norms, history, and experience with engagement efforts; (3) build trust and relationships and get commitments from formal and informal leadership; (4) collective self-determination is the responsibility and right of all community members; (5) partnering with the community is necessary to create change and improve health; (6) recognize and respect community cultures and other factors affecting diversity in designing and implementing approaches; (7) sustainability results from mobilizing community assets and developing capacities and resources; (8) be prepared to release control to the community and be flexible enough to meet its changing needs; and lastly, (9) community collaboration requires long-term commitment.

Over the past 30 years, guided by the Morehouse Model and incorporating the nine principles of CE, the HPRC has successfully implemented numerous projects and provided training or capacity-building technical assistance for almost 80 of Georgia's 159 counties. This chapter presents three case studies of funded prevention projects in both rural and micropolitan communities in central and west central Georgia. The lessons learned from these projects translate into effective strategies for engaging rural and micropolitan communities in health promotion and disease prevention activities.

Defining Metropolitan Statistical Areas, Micropolitan Statistical Areas, and Rural Communities

Community-level prevention projects or programs implemented in nonmetropolitan counties (rural and/or micropolitan counties), if successful in achieving outcomes and building collaboration, can have a tsunami effect in changing attitudes, knowledge, and behaviors beyond the target population. When scholars establish labels, it is generally for analytical purposes.[21] The US Office of Management and Budget (OMB) designates counties as Metropolitan, Micropolitan, or neither (see table 5.1).[22]

Defining rural areas is more complex than defining metropolitan and micropolitan statistical areas. Metropolitan and micropolitan areas are nationally delineated for statistical purposes. "Nonmetropolitan" is often used synonymously with "rural," and while there is overlap, these

Table 5.1 Definition of Geographical Areas

Classification	Definition	US number of areas defined by OMB
Metropolitan Statistical Area	A core-based statistical area associated with at least one urbanized area that has a population of at least 50,000. The Metropolitan Statistical Area comprises the central county or counties containing the core, plus adjacent outlying counties having a high degree of social and economic integration with the central county or counties as measured through commuting.	381 Metro SA
Micropolitan Statistical Area	A core-based statistical area associated with at least one urban cluster that has a population of at least 10,000 but less than 50,000. The Micropolitan Statistical Area comprises the central county or counties containing the core, plus adjacent outlying counties having a high degree of social and economic integration with the central county or counties as measured through commuting.	536 Micro SA
Completely rural[1]	These counties have no areas that are identified as urban and are home to less than 2.0% of the US population.	704 counties
Almost rural	In these counties, 33.1% of the population resides in urban areas, and 66.9% of the population resides in rural areas.	1,185 counties

Source: Ratcliffe, M., C. Burd, K. Holder, and A. Fields. 2016. *Defining Rural at the U.S. Bureau. Economic and Statistics Administration*, U.S. Census Bureau, census.gov.

Table 5.2 Case Studies

Case study	Project period	Funding source	Program location	OMB county classification
Case study A: Abstinence-Based Teenage Pregnancy Prevention Education Project	1997–2001	Federal	West central Georgia	Rural
Case Study B: HIV Prevention and Community Capacity Building Project	2015–20	Federal	County 1. Middle Georgia	Rural
			County 2. West central Georgia	Micropolitan
			County 3. West central Georgia	Micropolitan
			County 4. West central Georgia	Rural
			County 5. West central Georgia	Rural
Case Study C: Alcohol Abuse Prevention Project	2010–15	State	County 1. West central Georgia	Rural
			County 2. West central Georgia	Rural
			County 3. West central Georgia	Rural

geographic entities are not identical and should not be used interchangeably. The state of Georgia has 159 counties: 108 rural and 51 nonrural. According to the OMB classification, Georgia has eight micropolitan counties. However, the Georgia Department of Public Health Online Analytical Statistical Information System (OASIS) classification lists these counties as rural.[23] The case studies presented in this chapter will use the OMB county classification. Table 5.2 presents descriptive information on the three case studies.

Community Engagement and Mobilization

While funded mostly to work with youth in many of the projects, HPRC staff worked with parents and others in the community to transform them from unconsciously competent, not believing that they have the ability and right to advocate for their children, to consciously competent, empowered to advocate for change for their children and in their community.

To bring about lasting change and facilitate communications in communities imbued with a historical racial divide, the focus of our initial efforts was reducing at-risk behaviors among target youth, thereby addressing a problem that impacted the community across racial lines. With this agenda, in most instances, we were able to engage key stakeholders (e.g., county officials, school officials, law enforcement) in dialogue to discuss strategies to improve graduation rates, decrease delinquency, and address other community concerns. In most instances, our introduction to the community power structure was through the faith community or a community resident who had participated in one of our training sessions. Even with an introduction by a respected faith leader or a well-known community resident, the engagement process was often hampered by the stereotypes held by many rural White southerners of city folks and minorities. The primary strategies used to overcome negativity were persistence and not to take it personally.

On a parallel course, we worked with members of the minority communities to help them feel confident in their ability to advocate for their children and the needs in their community without hostility. In fact, in many parenting meetings and community trainings, we used part of a quote by Dr. Martin Luther King: "We fear each other because we do not know each other. We do not know each other because we do not communicate with each other."

In every Georgia county there is a countywide collaborative, the Family Connection Collaborative (FCC), initially created and funded by the state. Representatives of key county stakeholders are members of these collaboratives. The FCCs were created, at least in part, to address health disparities among at-risk populations. However, there was not significant representation from the minority population in many of our target counties. As part of our CE process in the micropolitan and rural counties in the case studies, we used the Community Engagement Continuum (CEC)[24] to increase the level of community involvement not only in the FCC but also in other community initiatives.

There are five phases in the CEC (see table 5.3). The purpose of the project and previous interactions with a community group determine the initial point of engagement. Outreach is the initial phase of the

Table 5.3 Community Engagement Continuum

	Increasing Level of Community Involvement, Impact, Trust, and Communication Flow			
Outreach	**Consult**	**Involve**	**Collaborate**	**Shared leadership**
Some community Involvement	More community involvement	Better community involvement	Community involvement	Strong bidirectional relationship
Communication flows from one to the other, to inform	Communication flows to the community and then back, answer seeking	Communication flows both ways, participatory form of communication	Communication flow is bidirectional	Final decision-making is at community level
Provides community with information	Gets information or feedback from the community	Involves more participation with community on issues	Forms partnerships with community on each aspect of project from development to solution	Entities have formed strong partnership structures
Entities coexist	Entities share information	Entities cooperate with each other	Entities form bidirectional communication channels	
Outcomes: optimally, establishes communication channels and channels for outreach	Outcomes: develops connections	Outcomes: visibility of partnership established with increased cooperation	Outcomes: partnership building, trust building	Outcomes: broader health outcomes affecting broader community; strong bidirectional trust built

Source: US Department of Health and Human Services. 2011. *Principles of Community Engagement*. 2nd ed. NIH Publication No. 11-7782. Washington, DC: US Department of Health and Human Services.

engagement process. This is consistent with step 1 in the Morehouse Model. In the start-up phase of most grant-funded programs, the primary grantee will be involved in community outreach. In this phase, there is limited community involvement and most of the communication is unidirectional. If there has been a lack of previous interactions with a community, or if there is a history of mistrust based on racial or cultural differences, the Outreach phase will be the most challenging to achieve. A failure to establish trust in the Outreach phase will delay progression through the CEC. It is in this phase that a champion or ambassador can facilitate the process. Because of the HPRC's relationship with the largest

African American religious organization in Georgia, the General Missionary Baptist Convention, and its work in nonmetropolitan communities, in most cases, we spent minimal time in the Outreach and Consult phases of the CEC. Progression along the other points of the CEC will be dependent on the purpose of the engagement and community resources.

There is a level of distrust, regardless of the racial/cultural persuasion of the outside entity, in most economically disadvantaged communities when approached about a new program. This can be more of a challenge in nonmicropolitan communities. The introduction and support of a champion or ambassador will facilitate the progress along the CEC to reach, in most cases, the Collaborate phase. The Shared Leadership phase is the most difficult point to achieve during most funding periods of a program. However, in most cases the HPRC, through its extensive work in south Georgia, has achieved the top levels (Collaborate and Shared Leadership phases) of CE on the CEC. It is difficult to state the amount of time it takes to move from one level to another on the CEC. There are many factors that can affect the progression to another level, such as resources, racial/cultural issues, mistrust, condescending attitudes, and perceived disrespect of community residents. Whether it is a new community or a community with which one has a history, it is helpful to review the CEC criteria and determine what level would be best for initiating CE activities. The CEC can be used as a checklist to assess progress in CE and the formation of a functioning collaborative.

As we worked to empower parents to become actively involved with the education of their children and to increase community readiness to become actively engaged in addressing community concerns, we also had to overcome negativity related to the HPRC's involvement in local concerns. It was easier in some instances to empower the minority community than to overcome the endemic racial and cultural barriers that stifled progress. When meeting with groups of African Americans, especially in rural communities, we provided a safe environment in which they could voice their feelings of frustration and helplessness. We conducted trainings that built their confidence to engage positively with those in power and become productive members of *any* community collaborative. We were successful in increasing collaboration and, to some extent, shared leadership in several of the communities over an extended period.

For example, in Case Study C, a project to address underage and binge drinking in a micropolitan community, the involvement of law enforcement was a challenge. To complete the needs assessment and monitor outcomes of environmental strategies, we needed local data from city and county law enforcement agencies. When the monthly meetings were moved to a local restaurant, attendance of both law and other key stakeholders increased. Because of improved collaboration, we gained timely access to alcohol arrest data and other related data from the law enforcement partners.

However, the disadvantage of morning or lunchtime meetings is that it limits participation of community residents. Representatives of social, health, education, law enforcement, and other agencies can attend daytime meetings as part of their workday. It is difficult for individuals who work in other areas or out of the county to attend a non-work-related meeting. Having collaborative meetings during the lunch hour limits participation of individuals working in other communities or far from the meeting location. A strategy that was effective in engaging community residents who wanted to participate with the collaborative was to schedule an evening meeting at least once a quarter. The trade-off was a decrease in attendance of official representatives. By the end of this five-year project, the local collaborative reached the Collaborate phase on the CEC. The community partners were involved with all aspects of the project, and communication was bidirectional with a high level of trust among the partners.

We incorporated the Cultural Competence Continuum (CCC) into our strategies to involve the White community and county leaders in addressing health and social disparities that impact the entire community, and this contributed to our success (see table 5.4). Cultural competence is a set of congruent behaviors, attitudes, and policies that come together in a system, agency, or individual and enable that system, agency, or individual to work effectively in cross-cultural situations.[25] The six points of the CCC were used to prioritize agencies and

Table 5.4 Six Points of the Cultural Competence Continuum

Cultural destructiveness	Cultural incapacity	Cultural blindness	Cultural pre-competence	Cultural competence	Cultural proficiency
Attitudes, policies, and practices destructive to other cultures; purposeful destruction and dehumanization of other cultures; assumption of cultural superiority; eradication of other cultures; or exploitation by dominant groups	Unintentional cultural destructiveness; a biased system, with a paternal attitude toward other groups; ignorance, fear of other groups and a culture; or discriminatory practices, lowering expectations and devaluating groups	The philosophy of being unbiased; the belief that culture, class, or color makes no difference, and that traditionally used approaches are universally applicable; a well-intentioned philosophy, but still an ethnocentric approach	The realization of one's own weakness in working with other cultures; implementation of training, assessment of needs, and use of diversity criteria when hired; desire for inclusion, commitment to civil rights; includes the danger of a false sense of accomplishment and tokenism	Acceptance and respect for differences; continual assessment of sensitivity to other cultures; expansion of knowledge; and hiring a diverse and unbiased staff	Cultures are held in high esteem; constant development of new approaches; seeking to add to knowledge base; advocates for cultural competency with all systems and organizations

Source: Stages and Levels of Cultural Competency Development, https://utahculturalalliance.files.wordpress.com/2015/10/stages_and_levels_of_cultural_competency_development.pdf.

institutions and evaluate individuals in our efforts to build collaboration in many of the target communities.

In our CE and development efforts to build sustaining support of projects, we learned to assess people and organizations according to the CCC. In many of our communities, we learned that some of the people who opposed our efforts and did not change were at the Cultural Destructiveness or the Cultural Incapacity points on the continuum. If not culturally destructive or incapable, they were at the point of Cultural Blindness. However, individuals and/or organizations at the blindness point were more accepting of constructive dialogue and trainings and moved along the continuum to Cultural Pre-competence. In some communities, we were successful in helping individuals, agencies, institutions, and organizations reach the fifth point, Cultural Competence. Getting the support of local government officials, school systems, and other key partners provided needed resources for the HPRC's success in implementing federally or state funded programs that resulted in building more diverse community collaboration with everybody at the table.

Institutional Readiness

Academic institutions by their very nature can be a barrier to effective CE. The agenda of the proposed CE is predicated on the goals, objectives, and timelines of the funded project. Academia's perception of superior knowledge of what is needed based on statistical data and ineffective communication with the target community can delay the progression on the CEC. One major stumbling block to forming mutually beneficial partnerships with a community is the concept "I know what you need." It is imperative that the leadership and staff are the "right fit" for working with a target community. Often when working with institutions of higher learning, CE activities are superficial or do not reach beyond the Outreach phase or Consult phase of the CEC. The goal of CE must be to increase the level of community involvement that results in sustainable collaborative efforts beyond the external funding. Project leadership must make ongoing assessments of staff interactions and performance with community partners using the guidelines of the

CEC and the Cultural Competence Continuum. The key to success is transparency and willingness to listen to the community. Failure to include the community at the beginning and throughout the project will result in less-than-optimal outcomes.

Case Studies

CASE STUDY A

Program Overview

Case Study A was a federally funded five-year abstinence-only after-school youth development program to address risk factors that contribute to the early initiation of sexual activity, poor attitudes toward education, and other negative behaviors among at-risk youth (see table 5.5). Prior to the initiation of this youth development project and the subsequent five-year program, expanding to an adjacent rural county, there was no teenage pregnancy prevention program in the county. Its goal was to implement an innovative program to increase protective factors, including parental involvement and community support of program activities. The objective of the program was to teach and support youth choice to remain abstinent until marriage. In response to the funder's guidelines, abstinence-only sex education was the sole contraceptive method that could be taught in the program. Because of the initial age of the participants, the abstinence-only curriculum was well received by this rural school system and parents. The program was offered to all fourth graders in the only school (K–8) in the

Table 5.5 Case Study A (Rural County)

Project	OMB county classification	County population	African American (%)	Persons in poverty[a] (%)
Case Study A: Abstinence-Based Teenage Pregnancy Prevention Education Project	Rural	2,962	60.7	35.2

Source: Georgia classification of rural and nonrural counties, Online Analytical Statistical Information System (OASIS), https://oasis.state.ga.us/oasis/webquery/qryPopulation.aspx.
[a] US Census Bureau QuickFacts: Georgia, https://www.census.gov/quickfacts/fact/table/ga.

county. As this cohort of 144 students progressed to the upper grades (sixth through eighth), adhering to the abstinence-only sex education mandate was a challenge, but the inclusion of other program activities (e.g., educational and cultural trips) minimized attrition from the program. Over the course of five years, economically disadvantaged youth were exposed to educational, social, and cultural events in other cities and states. The didactic abstinence-only curriculum was not as influential on sexual behavior as the extracurricular activities that exposed students to life outside of the third-poorest county in Georgia. Ninety-nine percent (143 out of 144) of the students remained in the program until they matriculated at a high school in another county.

Accomplishments

At the end of this five-year project, out of 144 youth who participated, only one pregnancy was documented. Other accomplishments included (1) active participation of parents in the parenting education program, (2) increased parental involvement and support of school activities, (3) improved community support and involvement in the project for the sustainability of select program components, and (4) improved interracial communication and inclusion of the minority population in local governance and the FCC. As explained earlier, the FCC is a partnership of several organizations working with families to research the needs of children and families in the community and find ways to address those needs. Prior to the project, African American representation on the FCC was minimal to nonexistent. By the end of the project, many members of the African American community attended local FCC meetings. Their participation influenced the FCC to include program data as part of its annual report. The impact of the teenage pregnancy prevention program is recognized on the local FCC website, referring to "the work of 'our partners' in the development and implementation of a comprehensive, holistic plan starting in 1992, and that the teenage pregnancy rate is now 42% lower."

Six years after the completion of the first program (1997–2001), a focus group was conducted by the HPRC. Ten young adults participated in the focus group. They credited the program with motivating many of the students to graduate from high school, attend college, or join the military. During the focus group, participants discussed the impact of the program and highlighted that only a few of the students had become pregnant and did not graduate from high school. Sixteen years later (2017), this poor rural county continued to have a teenage pregnancy rate (ages 15–17) below the state rate. The Georgia teenage pregnancy rate for this age group is 16.9; because County A had fewer than four pregnancies in this age group, a rate was not calculated.[26]

Challenges

The county in Case Study A, at the time of the project, was the third poorest of the state's 159 counties. The one public school was in poor physical condition; the student population was over 95 percent African American. The lack of constructive communication and collaboration between key community partners and the African American community was a major challenge for implementation and potential sustainability after federal funding. Some of the partners on the local FCC were the Department of Family and Children Services, Department of Public Health, Department of Juvenile Justice, Chamber of Commerce, individual businesses, Juvenile Court, Police Department, and Sheriff's Department. In this county, there was minimal representation of minorities in any of these organizations and agencies. The minority population in this county perceived that they did not have the skills or power to engage those in authority or to advocate for inclusion in the decision-making process in either the local government or the school system. Engaging the power structure was also a challenge; an assessment of some of the key partners placed them at the Cultural Destructiveness or Cultural Incapacity points on the CCC. It was more effective to begin with those partners who were higher on the continuum. Gaining the cooperation and to some extent the support of some of the key partners helped to begin the process of change in this community. There were some who would never accept diversity. However, the changing climate dissuaded overt hostility toward inclusion of the target population in the collaborative.

Lessons Learned

1. All parents, regardless of socioeconomic status, want the best for their children, but low-SES parents lack the skills or feel unable to advocate

for better educational opportunities for their children or to address concerns with the school system without appearing hostile. Parenting education workshops must include sessions to help parents develop self-efficacy to not only improve their parenting skills but also build their confidence to advocate for themselves and their children in a nonsupportive community environment.

2. Bridging the racial/cultural divide is not an overnight process. Overcoming decades of stereotypical interactions between White and minority populations requires patience and a plan of action. It is important that the plan of action is perceived not as "outside agitation" but as a process of improving the quality of life for all community residents.

3. It is important that the minority population feels empowered and competent before becoming a part of any collaborative or decision-making body.

4. Overcoming decades of racial separation to move to diversification in collaboration is a slow process, but it can be achieved if one uses the Cultural Competence Continuum as an assessment tool to improve dialogue between White and minority community residents. Accept the reality that there are some individuals who will never change or do not have the time or resources to invest in the effort; commit your energy and limited time to those at a higher level on the continuum to achieve positive results.

5. An outside agency can serve as a catalyst in the change process when dealing with decades of social injustice in racially and culturally divided communities. Initially when the HPRC became involved with this rural community, dialogue was mainly with the African American community. The only African American professionals in the community were teachers in the school system. In this small rural town, minorities were domestic workers, gardeners, or baggers in the only grocery store. After several years, a poultry plant opened in a neighboring county. Many of the residents were able to gain employment at the plant. This generated a new set of problems for single women with children. The long hours and lack of union representation created a hardship for these employees. Advocacy skills learned in dealing with issues at the school were transferrable to the employment environment. The women were empowered to address the injustices demonstrated by the White supervisors at the plant.

Table 5.6 Case Study B (Micropolitan and Rural Counties)

Project	OMB county classification[a]	County population	African American (%)	Persons in Poverty[b] (%)
Case Study B: HIV Prevention and Community Capacity Building Project	B.1. Rural	10,425	30.0	18.2
	B.2. Micropolitan	65,380	34.2	22.4
	B.3. Micropolitan	21,049	39.4	21.2
	B.4. Rural	18,217	9.6	11.2
	B.5. Rural	26,135	29.4	21.0

[a] "Rural" designation not based on population size; small incorporated community (county seat) with limited resources and less than 33% living in an incorporated community.
[b] US Census Bureau QuickFacts: Georgia, https://www.census.gov/quickfacts/fact/table/ga.

CASE STUDY B

Program Overview

Case Study B is a federally funded five-year (2015–20) HIV Capacity Building Initiative (HIV CBI) in partnership with a public health district composed of five networked county health departments (see table 5.6). In the target counties, there is a great need to enhance infrastructure to increase the capacity to implement, sustain, and improve effective substance abuse (SA), HIV, and viral hepatitis (VH) prevention services. The local health departments, which are funded through the state health department, provide HIV and VH counseling and testing, as well as sexually transmitted disease (STD) treatment. SA prevention services are funded by a different state agency and provided by the Department of Behavioral Health and Developmental Disabilities. There is a need for better communication, coordination, and leveraging of limited resources at both the state and local levels to address risk factors that contribute to behaviors resulting in negative life outcomes, such as SA, unplanned pregnancies and births, STDs, and HIV infection, especially among African Americans.

The overall goal of the MSM: HIV CBI is to build local capacity for delivering and sustaining evidence-based SA and HIV prevention services for the population of focus in the rural and micropolitan communities. Through a network of partners, the MSM: HIV CBI is providing culturally competent prevention information, educational workshops, and HIV testing and counseling for 3,773 adolescents and young adults, ages 13–24, regardless of sexual orientation and religious affiliation. The development of a continuum of services from prevention to treatment will require better communication at the local level, as well as implementation of organized community mobilization strategies to increase awareness of these problems and to gain the commitment of key stakeholders to work together to eliminate and/or reduce health inequities and health care disparities in the population of focus.

Accomplishments

Initially:
- Some community members had at least heard about local efforts, but knew little about them.
- Leadership and community members acknowledged that this issue is a concern in the community and that something must be done to address it.
- Community members had limited knowledge about the issue.
- There were limited resources that could be used for further efforts to address the issue.

By year 3:
- Most community members have at least basic knowledge of local efforts.
- Leadership plays a key role in planning, developing, and/or implementing new, modified, or increased efforts.
- The attitude in the community is "This is our responsibility," and some community members are involved in addressing the issue.
- Community members have basic knowledge about the issue and are aware that the issue occurs locally.
- Resources have been obtained and/or allocated to support further efforts to address this issue.

This progress supports the effectiveness of community mobilization strategies to increase the target communities' awareness of the issue and willingness to be involved with the proposed solutions to address SA and HIV infection.

There is increased collaboration among partners to provide SA and HIV prevention services for youth and young adults in the target counties.

Through monthly teleconferences, HPRC program staff and local health department nurse managers serve as the governing body to coordinate activities and data related to the project objectives. The Community Prevention Alliance Workgroup (CPAW), composed of HPRC staff, public health nurse managers, FCC coordinators, CBO representatives, and project evaluators, is an advisory collaborative that assists with outreach to the target communities and provides resources to achieve project objectives. Owing to limited resources, some of the public health nurse managers are administratively responsible for more than one local health department; hence, the use of teleconferences is an efficient method to increase participation and representation of all CPAW members.

Training needs of the community and local health department staff were identified through local focus groups, key informant interviews, and published data. In collaboration with the MSM Preventive Medicine Residency Program, the HPRC provided SA and HIV prevention training in the target communities. Partnership with a local college has increased the dissemination of prevention information to students and implementation of an evidence-based prevention program for students. There has been an increase in HIV, VH, and SA testing and referrals. To support collaboration, the MSM Mobile Health and Research Unit participates in local screening events in the target counties. Because the MSM mobile unit offers other health screenings, such as diabetes testing, there has been an increase in HIV testing. Especially in rural communities, there is still a stigma associated with being tested for HIV; the MSM Mobile Health and Research Unit allows residents to be covertly screened for HIV.

Challenges

The major challenge for the MSM: HIV CBI, after three years of implementation, is gaining access to the adolescent population through the local school systems. The alternative to reaching the adolescent target population is through local faith-based and CBOs. However, to reach the target number of youths, ages 13–18, partnership with local school systems was imperative. The CPAW was instrumental in creating this partnership. Members of the collaborative facilitated the process, and the HPRC participated in annual SA prevention education sessions held for juniors and seniors prior to proms, using the approved evidence-based SA prevention curriculum. With cooperating school systems, faith-based organizations, and CBOs, the project was able to reach its annual target numbers.

Another challenge is limited HIV referral resources and follow-up protocols in the health district. Owing to staffing shortage, outreach and information dissemination are primarily conducted at community screening events. The coordination of efforts through the CPAW has maximized limited resources.

Lessons Learned

1. Obtaining buy-in at the top of the organizational infrastructure is important to coordination received at the lower level. In this project, this moved slowly and required several telephone calls and in-person meetings to move from point A to point B. Again, CPAW members were crucial, especially in one micropolitan county, in obtaining support from the school system. Further, in rural and micropolitan counties, with limited public health manpower, the addition of new requirements and tasks, regardless of the need or benefit, may not be welcome. The blessings of the public health district director facilitated the process of cooperation.
2. Conducting a progress assessment and sharing community change is important to keep partners engaged in the project.
3. If there has not been progress, then further collaboration is needed to revise mobilization strategies. The key to revision is the inclusion of all relevant partners in the development of revised or new strategies.
4. The academic calendar of low-performing schools can serve as a barrier for the inclusion of nonacademic sessions. It is a priority of these schools to add academic sessions that increase students' performance on state standardized tests instead of nonacademic sessions. One strategy to facilitate a dialogue with local school administrators is to illustrate how HIV and other related health information will meet the requirements for state standards on health. Community advocates, including parents, will also help to open closed school doors.

Program Overview

Case Study C was a state-funded five-year contract to implement an alcohol prevention project (APP) to reduce binge and heavy drinking among young adults ages 18–25 in three rural counties in west central Georgia (see table 5.7). The primary and secondary goals of the APP were (1) to reduce binge drinking and heavy alcohol use and related consequences among young adults and (2) to reduce access to alcohol and binge drinking among children and adolescents ages 9–20. A major requirement of the contract was the development of a local community collaborative. The purpose of the local collaborative was to build capacity and infrastructure within an organization in a defined community and to work in partnership with other community stakeholders to execute strategies for achieving successful results.

The HPRC sought to train and provide technical assistance to community collaborative members in the use of the Strategic Prevention Framework (SPF)[27] to conduct a comprehensive needs assessment and build community capacity to address identified needs. The SPF uses a five-step planning process to guide the APP communities in the selection, implementation, and evaluation of effective, culturally appropriate, and sustainable prevention activities. The primary objective of the SPF process is to use findings from public health research along with evidence-based prevention programs to build capacity and sustainable prevention efforts at the local level. This, in turn, promotes resilience and decreases risk factors in individuals, families, and communities.

Table 5.7 Case Study C (Rural County)

Project	OMB county classification	County population	African American (%)	Persons in poverty[a] (%)
Case Study C: Alcohol Abuse Prevention Project	C.1. Rural	6,249	55.8	23.5
	C.2. Rural	10,425	30.0	18.2
	C.3. Rural	18,217	9.6	11.2
	Georgia	**10,429,378**	**32.2**	**14.9**

[a] US Census Bureau QuickFacts: Georgia, https://www.census.gov/quickfacts/fact/table/ga.

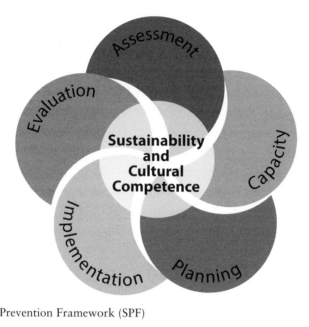

Strategic Prevention Framework (SPF)

Accomplishments

During the five-year contract period, considerable progress was made on achieving the project's goals because of active involvement of the local collaborative. A series of community activities were central. Two town hall meetings were held in two of the three target counties. They were projected to reach 80 community residents in both meetings. The actual number reached was 76, representing a cross section of residents, including government and nongovernment officials. Expert panelists shared information on issues related to alcohol use and abuse among youth and young adults in their respective communities. The panelists also engaged the audiences in dialogue regarding how accessibility to and promotion of alcohol products contribute to underage drinking and other negative consequences of excessive misuse of alcohol (driving under the influence [DUI]). Evaluations of the town hall meetings indicated increases in awareness and knowledge of the consequences and impact of underage drinking in their community.

As widespread awareness and knowledge increased, the CPAW found an increase in the number of recorded DUIs and arrests for drunkenness in counties with active participation of law enforcement in the collaborative. Evaluation contributed this trend to changes in attitude, knowledge, and willingness of local law enforcement to document underage drinking as a problem and not a "rite of passage." Parents and adults were held accountable and cited for providing alcohol at underage parties (e.g., graduation parties and proms). At collaborative meetings, there were open discussions on the causes of and solutions to disparities in arrests for DUIs and public drunkenness in their respective community.

COLLABORATION

Memoranda of understanding were established with multiple community partners, including local law enforcement, educational institutions, county governments, among others, not only to support the goals of the APP but also to provide resources to achieve project milestones. CPAW members disseminated SA prevention information and were involved in community events and other environmental strategies to mobilize the community to address binge and underage drinking in the target population. In two of three counties, traditional racial and cultural differences were minimized, and effective collaboration was achieved.

RESPONSIBLE BEVERAGE SERVER TRAINING

The HPRC developed a training video for on-site responsible beverage server training and educational packets to educate owners and employees on the Georgia law associated with selling alcohol to underage persons. In two of the counties, almost 85 percent of the owners and employees participated in the video training and received certificates and recognition from local chambers of commerce.

SOCIAL MARKETING CAMPAIGN

A multilevel social marketing campaign was launched that included media, billboards, posters, Facebook, newsletters, postcards, and palm cards placed in many businesses and disseminated at community events. These strategies were instrumental in increasing awareness.

The goal of this strategy was to gain the cooperation and support of local businesses that sold alcohol to limit the number of signs (no more than two) displayed in their windows or establishments. The support of the local chambers of commerce and recognition of those in compliance by the local media assisted in meeting this milestone.

Challenges

There were many challenges faced by the HPRC to achieve the contracted mandates of the APP. It was difficult to create a combined local collaborative that represented three adjacent counties. Further, innovative strategies were required to maintain the active participation of not only health, social, and educational representatives but also concerned community residents. The most effective strategy that increased involvement of law enforcement and other members was holding lunchtime meetings and providing food. To follow federal regulation, a training or transfer of technical information occurred during each of the luncheon meetings. The leadership of the local collaborative was shared among representatives of the three counties. Meetings were rotated, and the greatest number of collaborative members attended when a meeting was held in their specific county.

It was difficult to generate support and cooperation in one of the target counties owing to endemic racial and ethnic separation. The African American population was less than 10 percent, and most of the White population worked outside the county, commonly referred to as a bedroom county. It was difficult to conduct the required needs assessment because of racial distrust and the distances between houses outside of the small township. The minority population was clustered together in one neighborhood within the boundaries of the small township. The majority population was in control of the local government, school system, and law enforcement, and many of the potential key partners were either on the Cultural Destructiveness or Cultural Incapacity points on the Cultural Competence Continuum and were not receptive to our efforts. Without their support and involvement, our efforts were limited to working with local churches and organizations in the minority community, not countywide, as stipulated in our strategic plan. Fortunately, the FCC coordinator was an ambassador for our initiative. Near the end of the five-year project, he was instrumental in helping us bridge the communication gap. MSM-HPRC invited to participate in community events to disseminate information on alcohol abuse and SA.

Lessons Learned

1. Despite limitation in funding, it would have been better to establish local partnerships in each county. People are more concerned about issues that affect their local community and not those in other counties.
2. Do not spend limited time and resources trying to overcome decades of racial bigotry and mistrust. It is more effective to work with individuals and organizations that are willing to move beyond their comfort zone and engage with other races and/or cultures.
3. To be effective in CE and mobilization, the support and involvement of key community stakeholders (i.e., local government officials, faith community, school administrators, CBOs) are critical for success.
4. It is hard to generate support when a substance is legal (i.e. alcohol); therefore, the emphasis must be placed on the negative consequences of underage drinking and binge drinking (e.g., human and economic costs) to the community.
5. There must be a separation of powers and responsibilities to be effective. In the establishment of local partnerships, staff members play a significant role. As the leadership of the partnership becomes more effective, project staff must transition to a supportive role. If this does not occur, the local collaboration will not be sustained when contract funding expires.
6. There were several lessons learned when utilizing the SPF:
   a. *Assessment.*—Divide the labor among collaborative members and involve more members in the collection and analysis of community data. There was a greater buy-in of the results by collaborative members about their own community.
   b. *Capacity.*—Building relationships was important. It is important in building capacity that the intervention team is perceived not as competition but as a resource and asset. To engage local governments

(i.e., county or city officials, law enforcement) to address binge and underage drinking, the team must be clear about what it brings to the table.

c. *Planning.*—Inclusion is the key for developing a plan that will be accepted by all. When working with three distinct counties, strategic methodologies (county-specific work groups, teleconference meetings, planning retreat, etc.) must be utilized to ensure that plans will be accepted by respective collaborative members and the target community.

d. *Implementation.*—Allow stakeholders to select roles based on their expertise. It is crucial that all members feel that they have a part in the process, and they must be willing to recruit in their community to implement the proposed strategy or program.

e. *Evaluation.*—Utilize members with the expertise to collect, analyze, and report the data. An evaluation work group with representatives from each target county is an effective inclusion strategy. Members of the evaluation work group were involved in all aspects of the evaluation process (i.e., data collection, analysis, and generation of final evaluation report). HPRC staff and the external contract evaluator provided training and technical assistance to the evaluation work group to increase evaluation resources at the local level for sustainability after the state funding expired.

Summary

To successfully engage rural and micropolitan communities in health promotion and disease prevention activities, one must understand not only the principles of CE but also the culture and readiness to change of the target community. The Morehouse Model is predicated on the premise that the community should have a leadership role in the development, implementation, and oversight of programs. The role of the facilitating entity is to serve as a resource and catalyst for change. As the community becomes empowered, the role of the facilitating entity should lessen. The process of CE is not an overnight phenomenon and requires the inclusion of the decision-makers and the target population. Trust and accountability are key ingredients in building relationships in any environment. Because of the close-knit milieu of rural and micropolitan communities, word of mouth about a negative situation can derail a program. Many programs or projects have failed or had limited success because the professionals did not take the time to conduct a community assessment or spent limited resources on recalcitrant individuals resistant to change.

The case studies indicate that project staff must be willing to change and engage the community at all levels. If you are not part of the community, your actions must not be perceived as controversial or in competition with existing collaboratives or programs. Researchers and practitioners need to understand the cultural dynamics of specific groups and institutions to foster relationships, identify ways to effectively collaborate, and build respect and trust. This is an ongoing effort for all involved in the CE process.[28] Just because one is bringing resources into a community to address a concern, one should not think that this will eliminate or minimize all the barriers to developing supportive collaborations. Spending time to identify and cultivate ambassadors who will be assets for a project or program is well worth the effort. In the 30-year history of the HPRC's CE in mostly rural and micropolitan communities, we have had to learn that in some communities we could build bridges within the timeline of the funded project, and in others we had to accept the racial and cultural divide and work with the target population within the established community boundaries, hoping that one day doors of communication would open to facilitate inclusive collaboration.

References
1. Singh, G. K., and M. Siahpush. 2014. "Widening Rural-Urban Disparities in All-Cause Mortality and Mortality from Major Causes of Death in the USA, 1969–2009." *Journal of Urban Health* 91 (2): 272–92. doi:10.1007/s11524-013 -9847-2.

2. Ely, D. M., A. K. Driscoll, and T. J. Mathews. 2017. *Infant Mortality Rates in Rural and Urban Areas in the United States, 2014.* NCHS data brief, no. 285. Hyattsville, MD: National Center for Health Statistics.

3. Howard, G., D. O. Kleindorfer, M. Cushman, D. L. Long, A. Jasne, S. E. Judd, J. C. Higginbotham, and V. J. Howard. 2017. "Contributors to the Excess Stroke Mortality in Rural Areas in the United States." *Stroke* 48 (7): 1773–78. doi:10.1161 /STROKEAHA.117.017089.

4. Fontanella, C. A., D. L. Hiance-Steelesmith, G. S. Phillips, J. A. Bridge, N. Lester, H. A. Sweeney, and J. V. Campo. 2015. "Widening Rural-Urban Disparities in Youth Suicides, United States, 1996–2010." *JAMA Pediatrics* 169 (5): 466–73. doi:10.1001/jamapediatrics.2014.3561.

5. Singh, G. K., and M. Siahpush. 2009. "Widening Rural-Urban Disparities in Life Expectancy, U.S., 1969–2009." *American Journal of Preventive Medicine* 46 (2): e19–e29.

6. James, W., and J. S. Cossman. 2017. "Long-Term Trends in Black and White Mortality in the Rural United States: Evidence of a Race-Specific Rural Mortality Penalty." *Journal of Rural Health* 33 (1): 21–31. doi:10.1111/jrh.12181.

7. Alfero, C., T. Barnhart, D. Bertsch, S. Graff, D. Terry Hill, M. Ross, J. Schmidt, B. Slabach, and K. Sparks. 2013. *The Future of Rural Health: Why Rural Health Is Different*. Policy paper approved by the Rural Health Congress. Leawood, KS: National Rural Health Association.

8. Moy, E., et al. 2017. "Leading Causes of Death in Nonmetropolitan and Metropolitan Areas—United States, 1999–2014." *MMWR Surveillance Summaries* 66 (1): 1–8.

9. Cochran, G. T., R. J. Engel, V. J. Hruschak, and R. E. Tarter. 2017. "Prescription Opioid Misuse among Rural Community Pharmacy Patients: Pilot Study for Screening and Implications for Future Practice and Research." *Journal of Pharmacy Practice* 30 (5): 498–505. doi:10.1177/0897190016656673.

10. Keyes, K. M., M. Cerdá, J. E. Brady, J. R. Havens, and S. Sandro Galea. 2014. "Understanding the Rural-Urban Differences in Nonmedical Prescription Opioid Use and Abuse in the United States." *American Journal of Public Health* 104 (2): e52–e59. doi:10.2105/AJPH.2013.301709.

11. Mosher, H., Y. Zhou, A. L. Thurman, M. V. Sarrazin, and M. E. Ohl. 2017. "Trends in Hospitalization for Opioid Overdose among Rural Compared to Urban Residents of the United States, 2007–2014." *Journal of Hospital Medicine* 12 (11): 925–29. doi:10.12788/jhm.2793.

12. Dunn, K. E., F. S. Barrett, C. Yepez-Laubach, A. C. Meyer, B. J. Hruska, K. Petrush, S. Berman, S. C. Sigmon, M. Fingerhood, and G. E. Bigelow. 2016. "Opioid Overdose Experience, Risk Behaviors, and Knowledge in Drug Users from a Rural versus an Urban Setting." *Journal of Substance Abuse Treatment* 71:1–7.

13. Stein, E. M., K. P. Gennuso, D. C. Ugboaja, and P. L. Remington. 2017. "The Epidemic of Despair among White Americans: Trends in the Leading Causes of Premature Death, 1999–2015." *American Journal of Public Health* 107 (10): 1541–47. doi:10.2105/AJPH.2017.303941.

14. Hamilton, B. E., L. M. Rossen, and A. M. Branum. 2016. *Teen Birth Rates for Urban and Rural Areas in the United States, 2007–2015*. NCHS data brief, no. 264. Hyattsville, MD: National Center for Health Statistics.

15. Nandi, P., M. Kramer, and M. Kottke. 2018. "Changing Disparities in Teen Birth Rates and Repeat Birth Rates in Georgia: Implications for Teen Pregnancy Prevention." *Contraception* 99 (3): 175–78. doi:10.1016/j.contraception.2018.11.007.

16. Jacob Arriola, K. R., et al. 2016. "Promoting Policy and Environmental Change in Faith-Based Organizations: Outcome Evaluation of a Mini-Grants Program." *Health Promotion Practice* 17 (1): 146–55. doi:10.1177/1524839915613027.

17. Sullivan, G., et al. 2014. "Building Partnerships with Rural Arkansas Faith Communities to Promote Veterans' Mental Health: Lessons Learned." *Progress in Community Health Partnerships* 8 (1): 11–19. doi:10.1353/cpr.2014.0004.

18. Bryant, K., T. Moore, N. Willis, and K. Hadden. 2015. "Development of a Faith-Based Stress Management Intervention in a Rural African American Community." *Progress in Community Health Partnerships* 9 (3): 423–30. doi:10.1353/cpr.2015.0060.

19. Schoenberg, N. E., C. R. Studts, B. J. Shelton, M. Liu, R. Clayton, J. B. Bispo, N. Fields, M. Dignan, and T. Cooper. 2016. "A Randomized Controlled Trial of a Faith-Placed, Lay Health Advisor Delivered Smoking Cessation Intervention for Rural Residents." *Preventive Medicine Reports* 3:317–23. doi:10.1016/j.pmedr.2016.03.006.

20. Centers for Disease Control and Prevention. 1997. *Principles of Community Engagement.* 1st ed., 59. Atlanta: CDC/ASTDR Committee on Community Engagement.

21. Flora, C. B., and J. L. Flora. 2013. *Rural Communities: Legacy and Change.* 4th ed. Boulder, CO: Westview.

22. "2010 Standards for Delineating Metropolitan and Micropolitan Statistical Areas." https://www.federalregister.gov/documents/2010/06/28/2010-15605.

23. "Population Statistics." Georgia Department of Public Health, Office of Health Indicators for Planning. https://oasis.state.ga.us/oasis/webquery/qryPopulation.aspx.

24. US Department of Health and Human Services. 2011. *Principles of Community Engagement.* 2nd ed. NIH Publication No. 11-7782. Washington, DC: US Department of Health and Human Services.

25. Cross, T. L. 1988. "Cultural Competence Continuum." *Focal Point.* Portland, OR: Portland State University.

26. "Population Statistics." Georgia Department of Public Health, Office of Health Indicators for Planning. https://oasis.state.ga.us/oasis/webquery/qryPopulation.aspx.

27. Substance Abuse and Mental Health Services Administration. 2019. *A Guide to SAMHSA's Strategic Prevention Framework.* https://www.samhsa.gov/sites/default/files/dtac/ccptoolkit/samhsa-strategic-prevention-framework-guide.pdf.

28. Centers for Disease Control and Prevention. 1997. *Principles of Community Engagement.* 1st ed., 9. Atlanta: CDC/ASTDR Committee on Community Engagement.

six

Educational and Leadership Development— for Communities, by Communities

The Strategic Engagement of Community Health Workers

TRUE TO its crosscutting theme of community- and patient-centric re-search, education, clinical care, and service, Morehouse School of Medicine (MSM) has prioritized the education, employment, and leadership of neighborhood residents trained as community health workers (CHW). According to the American Public Health Association, a CHW is a "frontline public health worker who is a trusted member and/or has an unusually close understanding of the community served (Step 1 in the Morehouse Model for Community Engagement). This trusting relationship enables the worker to serve as a liaison/link/intermediary between health/social services and the community to facilitate access to services and improve the quality and cultural competence of service delivery."[1] In the context of advancing equity strategies for health disparity populations (defined by location, race/ethnicity, gender, health status, or any combination), MSM has strategically and intentionally prioritized particular eligibility criteria for CHWs that it has enlisted over time. Equally, if not more important than training and skills, is living and leading in and/or being a representative of the health disparity population served through the research or health promotion intervention. These criteria build and foster the trust and relationships between community residents and academics historically fractured or broken by social, political, or civil exploitation.

CHWs at MSM have supported a broad array of research projects, health initiatives, and other policy, systems, and environmental change approach strategies. Areas of focus have included, but are not limited to, diabetes, cardiovascular health, cancer, primary care prevention strategies, and linkages to patient-centered medical homes (PCMHs). The sections that follow demonstrate the integration of CHWs as leaders in the planning, implementation, and assessment of research, educational, and clinical pillars of MSM.

Lay Health Worker—Breast and Cervical Cancer Intervention

Blumenthal et al.[2] were among the first investigators to describe the role of lay health workers (LHWs) in recruitment and delivery of a longitudinal breast and cervical cancer prevention educational trial among low-income Black women. LHWs recruited from the same communities as intervention participants were trained over a 10-week period on interviewing skills and intervention delivery. The intervention was conducted in homes and consisted of educational materials; interactive discussions on breast and cervical cancer; screening tests, including Pap smears, clinical exams, self-exams, and mammography; and other women's health information. This community-centered recruitment strategy was more successful when compared to recruitment from the patient registry of a primary health care center. This success, despite challenges detailed elsewhere, was attributed to LHWs and other project staff in community organizations, meetings, and activities that capitalized on face-to-face interactions, existing social networks, and working with community leaders.

Atlanta Choice Neighborhoods

MSM's Department of Community Health and Preventive Medicine serves as the medical lead for the Atlanta Choice Neighborhoods Initiative. Nationally, Choice Neighborhoods is funded through a US

Department of Housing and Urban Development initiative designed to transform distressed neighborhoods into thriving communities with quality, affordable housing and amenities that meet the needs of their residents.[3] The Atlanta Housing Authority (AHA) Choice Neighborhood priority communities include the former University Homes public housing project and three surrounding neighborhoods on the city's west side: Vine City, Ashview Heights, and the Atlanta University Center neighborhood (collectively known as the University Choice Neighborhood). MSM's CHW leadership efforts include the training and deployment of CHW care coordinators to assist clients referred by AHA case managers in the coordination of care with our medical partners (Morehouse Health Care, Neighborhood Union Public Health Clinic, Family Health Centers of Georgia). Our health partners provide resources, home visits, and mental health services to assess household health care needs and assist residents in linkages to health care.

Health 360x

Health 360x is a mobile health application and social platform that integrates self-monitoring and decision support for preventive health developed by the MSM Clinical Research Center. Health coaches (equivalent to CHWs) were trained on the Health 360x curriculum, adapted from the American Association of Diabetes Educators (AADE). Community leaders from partner churches served as health coaches, promoting participation as health coaches or study participants.[4-6] Independent physician practice members of the MSM Community Physicians Network were invited to join the study, with each enlisted practice identifying a physician champion and a health coach within the practice. The health coaches were trained and certified using a program designed by the AADE for staff at the point of care of diabetes. Additional health coach training was provided on the use of the structured goal-setting and counseling tool, as well as technical training for web access to assist study participants. All diabetic patients in each practice were identified using the ICD-10 codes for diabetes mellitus. The intervention included weekly coaching with 15–20 study participants for 12 weeks, as well as facilitation of online peer networking. Participants were encouraged to log on to the website and join informal peer support groups. Blood pressure, physical activity, and blood glucose showed significant improvement at 12 weeks and 12 months compared to baseline.

Educational Program to Increase Colorectal Cancer Screening

CHWs were deployed at each phase of a 10-year community-based participatory research process for research, implementation, and adaptation of an intervention designed to increase colorectal cancer screening among African American men and women ages 50 and older—from CBPR intervention to implementation across the state of Georgia.[7] First, from 2002 to 2008, three salaried CHWs played a central role in the conduct of a randomized controlled community intervention trial through recruitment of participants, administration of questionnaires, supporting the delivery of a group education intervention, and conducting participant follow-up. As detailed in chapter 3, the intervention ultimately enrolled randomized participants in one of three interventions (one-on-one education, group education, and reducing out-of-pocket costs). The group education model was found to be the most efficacious at six months following the intervention, with colorectal cancer screening rate of twice those in the control group. Second, CHWs helped deliver the intervention and follow up with participants in the expansion of the intervention to 17 senior centers, where it was proven to be as effective in practice as in the research project.[8] Third, CHW facilitators recruited by five of the state's publicly funded cancer coalitions were trained throughout the state to deliver the intervention in a dissemination and implementation project beginning in 2010.[8] A grant from the National Cancer Institute (NCI) enabled the testing and adaptation of EPICS at 20 sites around the country.[9] In this project, the intervention is being tested under varying circumstances to identify the best approach to training the health educators and CHWs.[10]

Community Intervention Trial (2002–2008)
- 369 African Americans, ≥50 years of age
- Randomized to control, one-on-one education, group education, or reduced out-of-pocket costs
- Post-intervention CRC screening: 17.7%; controls: 33.9%; small group education (p = 0.039): 25.4%; one-on-one education (p = ns); and 22.2% reduced out-of-pocket cost groups (p = ns)

Local Practice Demonstration (2009–2010)
- Small group education
- 331 African Americans, ≥50 years of age
- Post-intervention screening: 37.3%: 33.8% stated that they had appointments for screening or intended
- Performed at least as well in practice as it did in the community intervention trial

State Practice Demonstration (2010)
- Small group education
- 900 African Americans, ≥50 years of age (targeted)
- Results pending

National Dissemination and Implementation (2011)
- R01 grant application/sustainability plan
- 7,200 African Americans, ≥50 years of age (targeted)
- Results pending

Educational Program to Increase Colorectal Cancer Screening Intervention Phases

The ABCD Community Intervention Pilot Project

The MSM National Center for Primary Care tested the effectiveness of CHWs to educate their peers about cardiovascular disease (CVD) and risk reduction.[11] The intervention utilized the American Diabetes Association and the National Diabetes Education Program ABC approach (glycated hemoglobin A1c, blood pressure, cholesterol) for identifying and controlling the leading indicators of CVD risk. Prioritizing the unique contextual factors of low-income African Americans, a D factor, for depression, was added owing to this disorder's predictiveness for CVD risk, control of diabetes, and lack of inclusion in similar interventions. CHWs participated in a 16-hour training session and subsequently delivered a six-week tailored educational program with counseling sessions and demonstrations. The control group received a weekly lecture by clinical experts. The CHW active learning intervention was more effective than lectures by clinical experts in increasing the knowledge of CVD risk among African Americans.

Peer-to-Peer Community Health Workers to Improve Heart Health

The Clinical Research Center implemented a peer-to-peer training to build the capacity of CHWs to deliver cardiovascular health education to African American women, who disproportionately experience poorer heart health risk factors, higher morbidity, and mortality.[12] CHWs were recruited from community-based organizations, faith-based organizations, and organizations with a focus on CVD prevention or women's health. Experienced CHWs were also invited. The training was designed to increase knowledge of heart healthy habits, enhance the core competencies of CHWs who predominantly serve African American females, and build a replicable and sustainable CHW training model for community organizations to address heart health using CHWs as health educators. A Learning Circle approach blending web-based, self-directed learning and in-person peer coaching was employed. CHWs demonstrated increased heart health knowledge, increased training satisfaction, and 100% training retention. CHWs also initiated and subsequently delivered 122 person-hours of community heart health education and CHW training in their local communities.

Center of Excellence on Health Disparities

The National Institutes of Health funded the MSM Center of Excellence on Health Disparities (CEHD), with an emphasis on the reduction of health disparities in vulnerable African American families and communities. The CEHD funded research projects centered on (1) the impact of secondhand smoke on children, (2) HIV/AIDS risk reduction among female social offenders reentering communities from incarceration, and (3) the impact of parent education on child and adolescent development through a Smart and Secure Children Initiative.[13–14] The center included a CE core, capitalizing on the successful CBPR governance of the MSM Prevention Research Center (PRC) Community Coalition Board (CCB), through which research and related health promotion strategies are led or co-created by community residents in 31 census tracts representing four neighborhood planning units (see chap. 5 for details on the MSM PRC and CCB governance model).[15–16] Through the CE core funding, the MSM PRC coalition board chair (a community leader), a CCB member, and a community resident with the partner community were strategically hired (one consultant and full-time CHWs). Their engagement elevated the community credibility, relevance, and resonance of the research and created opportunities for neighborhood resident education and research engagement. CHWs developed and conducted workshops consisting of nationally and locally relevant educational overviews on the significance of PCMHs and linkage with health insurance navigators at community meetings. Subsequently, full-length one-hour workshops were conducted through their partnerships with local libraries, neighborhood associations, and other civic organizations that served as workshop host sites. Presentations and interactive sessions included CHW-developed pamphlets detailing PCMH-designated organizations in the neighborhood toward community-clinical linkages for health care.

Racial and Ethnic Approaches to Community Health (REACH)

The MSM REACH project was funded by the Centers for Disease Control and Prevention. The partners in this comprehensive implementation grant were the MSM PRC, the CCB, the Satcher Health Leadership Institute, Georgia State University, and the National Center for Primary Care. It employed an evidence-based and culturally tailored model to address CVD and diabetes risk through community-based policy, systems, and environmental approaches.[17–18] Application for this grant was in direct response to a community-led needs assessment conducted by the MSM CCB in collaboration with neighborhood residents in 31 census tracts characterized by high rates of often co-occurring CVD and diabetes.

Eight strategically hired CHWs were central to the implementation of all approaches. The community-clinical linkages component (iADAPT 2.0) was designed to increase chronic disease self-management and prevention by promoting access to PCMHs and nonphysician care teams incorporating CHWs. Four CHWs supported or led three-day workshops with over 300 CHWs and community residents to promote chronic disease self-management. iADAPT 2.0 provided both CHWs and community residents virtual resources through the iADAPT website and a physical resource center with a computer work room and information to help CHWs continue assisting patients and residents.

Four CHWs were integral to the project's Healthy Corner Store Initiative (HCSI). The HCSI was identified as an evidence-based intervention that could be culturally tailored and used to address the food desert themes that emerged from the community health needs assessment, a community-identified determinant of diabetes, high blood pressure, and overweight/obesity. CHWs conducted an environmental scan of corner stores in 31 census tracts, supported the conduct of surveys among corner store patrons to identify buying patterns and preferences for health food options, and worked with corner store owners to establish relationship supports and agreements associated with increasing their capacity to carry, market, and promote healthy foods. Their leadership resulted in 11 corner stores being enlisted in the Healthy Corner Store Network.[18]

Patient-Centered Medical Home and Neighborhood Project

The MSM Patient-Centered Medical Home and Neighborhood Project, funded in 2014 by the Optum Foundation, was designed to implement an integrated approach to improve outcomes and decrease costs for a discrete population of patients with multiple health risk factors and comorbidities.[19] The implementation approach was led by the MSM Department of Family Medicine in coordination with MSM's array of population health, community outreach, and primary/specialty care assets in East Point, Georgia. Identified patients participated in an intervention (minimum of 90 days) consisting of four home visits by CHWs, at least one clinic visit with patients' primary care physician, an individualized plan of care toward condition self-care management, and linkages to community supports and CE activities. The community supports and engagement component was led by the PRC through a community advisory group, community support liaisons, facilitators of community linkages, and CHWs. The care coordination team included a project director, a physician champion, family practice residents, four CHWs, a community support and engagement specialist, a data analyst, a data coordinator, a nurse care manager, and a licensed clinical social worker; they met for at least two hours every Friday to discuss the needs of patients who were scheduled to have home visits that week and patients who received home visits the week prior.

The High School Community Health Worker Program

MSM scaled its CHW efforts toward addressing the crosscutting priorities of fostering future learners and leaders in health disparity communities and building community-engaged initiatives that foster neighborhood leadership. The program serves students ages 15–18 who are at least rising sophomores. The objectives of the High School CHW (HS CHW) program are to

- increase the number of trained student CHWs to assist with community health programs in underserved communities;
- provide a health career pipeline program and mentorship for underserved students;
- support and promote the CHW field;
- promote health education and health literacy in schools and community; and
- assist trained HS CHWs with the design and implementation of school-based and community-based health initiatives.

The HS CHW training is 140 hours, with two weeks (70 hours) of didactic instruction followed by 70 hours of field instruction and additional hours of continuing education opportunities. Continuing education occurs bimonthly (twice per month) over 12 months and includes but is not limited to teleconferences, face-to-face instruction, and workshops. In 2018, the program launched an online training consisting of 18 modules covering CHW core competencies, including student support in critical thinking, decision-making, and communication skills.[20] Each module consists of a welcome video, pre-learning quiz, readings, activities, assignments, and a post-learning quiz. Students create videos and presentations and interact with other students and community members. Upon completion of all the modules, students are able to download a certificate of completion. This certificate may be used toward school community service hours, to apply for CHW and similarly skilled jobs, or as part of their college applications and the first step toward a health career. Participating students are afforded opportunities to interact with their peers by exchanging their beliefs, ideas, and thoughts through digital stories, presentations, and participation in group discussions. This training program, recognized and featured by the American Association of Medical Colleges,[21] will introduce a new cadre of emerging adults to the field of community health and turn them into workers able to take an active role in the health and wellness of their communities.

Training and Deployment of Community-Engaged Faculty, Students, and Staff

Originally a two-year educational program in the basic medical sciences, MSM now confers doctor of medicine (MD), doctor of philosophy in biomedical sciences (PhD), master of public health (MPH), master of science in biomedical research (MSBR), master of science in biomedical technology (MSBT), master of science in clinical research (MSCR), and master of science in medical sciences (MSMS) degrees. Among these, five have integrated required or elective courses in CE in research, training, and practice.

The Doctor of Medicine Community Health Course

To meet the growing needs of communities with increased chronic conditions, decreased health care access, and changing sociocultural environments, community-oriented physicians equipped with the skills to attend to the health of underserved populations are paramount. The MSM Community Health Course (CHC) was designed to develop community-oriented physicians with the empathy and tools needed to care for diverse populations who can address the social determinants of health to achieve health equity. The CHC is a required course that provides didactic and hands-on instruction to all first-year medical students with the guidance of over 20 interprofessional faculty members with backgrounds in medicine, public health, patient advocacy, policy, academia, and federal service. Students are organized into groups and assigned to community organizations for a half-day per week throughout the year (two semesters from August to April). Among projects to which students have been assigned are those serving urban youth, seniors, and homeless persons in settings that include elementary schools, afterschool programs, senior residential facilities, and a homeless shelter for women and children. These organizations partner with MSM students to complete community needs and assets assessments in the fall semester and to develop, implement, and evaluate interventions in the spring semester. Students who excel in the CHC can also pursue honors in community service. Other community assignments for students include placement in community practices or clinics in the first-year preceptorship program and the third-year family medicine pediatrics or rural primary care clerkships. Additional information about this course is provided in chapter 2.

Master of Public Health Program

The MPH program at MSM was established in 1995 to address the shortage of underrepresented minorities in leadership positions in the field of public health. MSM-trained public health professionals are prepared for careers that will engage them in addressing and protecting the health of people of color, minorities, and underserved communities that are disproportionately affected by preventable chronic conditions and illnesses. The MPH curriculum ensures that all MSM MPH degree recipients are proficient in the community-focused work that undergirds the social mission of the institution while still meeting or exceeding the accreditation standards set forth by the Council on Education for Public Health (CEPH). The program was accredited initially in 1999 by CEPH, making it the first accredited MPH program at a historically Black college or university.

The MPH program focuses on providing unique opportunities for students to become engaged in CE/CBPR, student-directed learning, problem-solving, and the development of skills and competencies essential to the practice of public health. MSM is located within the historic West End community in Atlanta. Courses equip students with foundational knowledge and concepts essential for them to optimally understand the needs of the populations they serve. The community-focused coursework and required community service hours ensure that the program has a strong service learning component. Students spend the equivalent of three months with a community agency in their practicum. Among the goals of the program is to provide community health assessments, community service, and ultimately measurable improvement.

The Master of Science in Medical Sciences (MSMS) Community Assessment and Health Program Course

The MSMS program is a two-year, nonthesis degree that includes graduate coursework in biochemistry, anatomy and physiology, neurobiology, medical microbiology, medical pharmacology, biomedical genetics, epidemiology, and biostatistics. It is designed to improve performance and standardized test scores. Beyond these nationally recognized program features is a course on the Community Assessment and Health Program (GEBS 548). GEBS 548 is designed to provide students with the knowledge and skills central to assessing and organizing communities for health promotion interventions. Students work as teams in select communities and engage in fact-finding activities that lead to the development of grant proposals based on community assessments that inform responsive implementation strategies. These experiences are designed to provide exposure to real-time CE collaboration toward program planning in response to identified priorities, including the development of goals and objectives and a logic model for the proposed intervention with an evaluation component.

The Master of Science in Clinical Research Community Engagement and Health Disparities in Clinical and Translational Research Course

Current translational research has progressed beyond the traditional bench to the bedside and now includes translating scientific evidence into clinical practice and extending further into community settings. This development has been a dynamic progression involving patient, physician, community, and academic organizational structures informed by translational strategies.[9] The Atlanta Clinical and Translational Science Institute (funded 2007–17) and the subsequently funded Georgia Clinical and Translational Science Alliance (funded 2017–22) were and continue to be interinstitutional collaborations between Emory University, MSM, and the Georgia Institute of Technology. The Georgia CTSA Community Engagement (CE) Programs were designed to advance the art, science, and practice of community-engaged clinical and translational research that is broadly disseminated to and adapted in communities of residents/patients and practice (clinical and research leaders, among others) toward improved population health. The Community Engagement and Health Disparities in Clinical and Translational Research (CEHCTR) course was developed by the CE program in collaboration with other ACTSI cores to support junior faculty, predoctoral (medical, doctoral, or PharmD students) or postdoctoral (resident and fellow physicians, PhD postdocs, PharmD residents), who want to become successful clinical and translational researchers. The course, a requirement for all MSCR students, across partner institutions, Is an introduction to the concepts, methods, and issues involved in community-engaged research.

The core competencies of the CEHCTR course were developed by the CE Research Steering Committee Competency Work Group in collaboration with Georgia CTSA CE faculty and community representatives toward integration into the translational research paradigm. The course was and continues to be governed by the CE program's Community Steering Board, adopted from the MSM PRC CCB model, with most of its members from the community, rather than from partner academic institutions. The course's primary texts were written and edited by MSM and Emory University faculty leaders in CE research.[19, 22, 23]

Special emphasis is given to social and behavioral science concepts and methods, principles and historical roots of CE, clinical and translational research partnerships, multidisciplinary research collaborations, ethical issues, and practical considerations in planning, implementing, evaluating, and disseminating community-engaged research. Case studies and course projects are shaped to accommodate students with diverse interests in health disparities, communities, and/or translational research. Students are assumed to have a general research and clinical background, but the course emphasizes research theory and concepts with the goal of encouraging thoughtful and effective community-based research collaborations. Unique to the course are lectures, panels, and workshops delivered by research agency and community leaders advising on the pedagogy and real-time processes, outcomes, and lessons learned in the conduct of CE. No other required, for-credit course in CE for MSCR students has been identified, across the national CTSA network.

Elective Courses and Competitive or Voluntary Leadership
Bridges to Health Equity Course

This course, with original support by the National Institutes for Minority Health and Health Disparities, is designed to help learners understand the ways that individual, social, institutional, and historical injustices impact health disparities and to provide instruction in the concepts, methods, key issues, and research tools necessary for conducting health equity research, with emphasis on the research frameworks applicable to understanding and intervening in the social determinants of health to achieve health equity. The course provides a platform for interdisciplinary discourse on the impact of the intersection of race/ethnicity, socioeconomic status, gender, sexuality, and environment on how people grow, live, work, and age.

There are currently three iterations of the Bridges to Health Equity course. The first, delivered online, is offered over a 12-week semester to graduate students across all MSM academic programs, including Graduate Education in Biomedical Sciences and Graduate Education in Public Health (MPH). The second iteration is a four-week Health Equity resident rotation, which is delivered as an in-person/online hybrid for MSM residents across all the residency programs. We have also tailored a third four-session iteration of the course that has been offered to high school and college students who participate in the MSM summer programs. The course has also been selected as 1 of 10 priority foundational courses for the recently funded Massive Open Online Courses (MOOCs) across all Georgia CTSA partner academic institutions (Emory University, Georgia State University, MSM, and the University of Georgia).

Community Health Advanced by Medical Practice Superstars

The Community Health Advanced by Medical Practice Superstars (CHAMPS) program, funded by the US Health Resources and Services Administration to the MSM Department of Medicine, trains and supports primary care champions who will be equipped and empowered to lead health care transformation and teaching in urban and rural community-based settings (Atlanta metropolitan areas, federally qualified health centers).[24] This program, designed for early and mid-career physicians and physician assistants, functions to (1) develop leadership capacity in health care transformation for primary care professionals, (2) increase integrated and coordinated care services within and between care settings, (3) improve the quality of care in health care organizations, and (4) increase patient access to care. Selected fellows

- earn CME through online course instruction;
- engage in practical leadership and quality improvement instruction through virtual clinic site visits;
- participate in monthly coaching sessions and technical assistance;

- complete a health care transformation project with a focus on one of the three Department of Health and Human Services priorities—childhood obesity, mental health, and opioid abuse;
- build leadership skills that strengthen change processes in organizations; and
- become part of a team to coach and mentor future CHAMPS fellows.

The Health Equity for All Lives Clinic

The MSM student-run clinic Health Equity for All Lives (HEAL) was established in 2011 by members of the 2014 medical student class.[25] Guided by MSM Department of Family Medicine faculty and advisors, its purpose is to serve people of color and other underserved populations in Georgia. Beginning with community primary care clinics for scheduled patients once a month, it has now expanded to two clinics a month, as well as sites in rural Georgia. Clinic co-directors are medical students supported by translators for Spanish-speaking patients. This voluntary experience provides community-engaged clinical experience, leadership, and teaching skills for the medical students who co-direct it. These clinics train students in delivery of free primary care services, including medical, dental, laboratory, subsidized medications, and specialty referral. The Rural MSM HEAL on Wheels mobile clinic, a collaboration with the MSM Clinical Research Center, provides medical screenings (blood pressure, blood sugar, HIV, and hepatitis C) and educational materials.

The Medical Student Summer Research Experience

The Medical Student Summer Research Experience offers competitively selected rising second-year MSM medical student applicants the opportunity to participate in scientific research (from basic laboratory to social/behavioral) with nationally renowned researchers, mentors, and clinical scientists at their home institution. This paid summer program is designed to increase interest and support toward the development and preparation of careers in academic medicine that align with the institutional mission of serving the underserved and advancing health equity. Initially focused primarily on biomedical research experiences, infusion of the Summer Scholars in the Community (SSiC) expands the program through broadened understanding and expertise in working with communities. SSiC scholars participate in weekly didactic and experiential activities addressing community health skills, social determinants of health and health equity sensitivity, and related response strategies. They also participate in scheduled activities designed to advance skills in community needs assessments. All students work toward the preparation and submission of a research abstract and presentation at a professional organization or society meeting at the end of the program.

Fostering Community Leadership in Research Practice and Policy
Community Understanding of Research: Flipping the Script

The MSM PRC developed and delivers the Understanding of Research trainings in all research partner communities. The purpose of the "Understanding Research Methods—Flipping the Script" trainings is to educate and facilitate a dialogue with community members toward understanding the importance of their involvement, critical perspectives, and leadership as research partners, rather than solely participants. A CBPR approach was employed to develop a culturally tailored two-hour training, with content, logistics, and recruitment led by a team composed of the MSM PRC. CHWs residing in research partner communities in 31 census tracts led recruitment of trainings and content development. To sustain the theme of flipping the script, the research teams were charged with developing an interactive, nonacademic depiction of their projects, designed to increase research interest and recruitment, rather than traditional podium or PowerPoint presentations. Resulting "presentations" included interactive skits, games, demonstrations, and videos. The foundation of the trainings advised the development of an expanded CBPR curriculum with modules that include research ethics, CE research (defined), evaluation, building and sustaining community-academic research partnerships, and collaborative dissemination of community-engaged research.[26]

Satcher Community Health Leadership Programs

The MSM Satcher Health Leadership Institute (SHLI) has been intentional in its efforts to train, equip, and empower community residents to lead or equitably collaborate in initiatives designed to promote thriving communities. The SHLI mission is to "develop a diverse group of exceptional health leaders, advance and support comprehensive health system strategies, and actively promote policies and practices that will reduce and ultimately eliminate disparities in health."[27] Three signature programs designed for community leaders include the Smart and Secure Children Program, the Mayor's Healthy Communities Initiative, and the Community Health Leadership Program (CHLP). Since 2009, SHLI Signature Leadership Programs have engaged over 800 diverse learners across 26 states and are detailed below.

Smart and Secure Children Parenting

SHLI's Smart and Secure Children Parenting Leadership Program (SSC) is designed with and for members of disparate targeted communities. The program focuses on transforming parents and guardians within vulnerable health disparity populations into community leaders who can learn and lead in development of their children and peers. SSC is a product of the SHLI Neighborhood Healthy Child Development project, which was designed with parents through a community participatory study to increase quality parenting and to strengthen vulnerable families raising children 0–5 years old who may have been exposed to negative childhood experiences. The program trains and deploys parents to lead parenting education sessions that will transform parenting culture and provide communal social support. SSC parenting sessions are evaluated to assess direct impacts on quality parenting, child behavior, and preschool ability.[14–16]

The SSC has evolved over time to include two distinct arms, the Collaborative Action for Child Equity (CACE) and Using Quality Parenting to Address Health Inequities. The vision of CACE is to reduce disparities in health and promote well-being and school readiness for children ages 0–5. It is also designed to contribute to bridging early childhood policy and program gaps for disparate and vulnerable families through healthy children who are school ready at age 5. CACE was funded through the MSM Transdisciplinary Collaborative Center (National Institutes of Health) to engage nine states. These include the CDC-designated Racial and Ethnic Health Disparities Action Institute states[15] (Maryland, Minnesota, Missouri, Oregon, and Texas) and Department of Health and Human Services Region IV states (South Carolina, North Carolina, Georgia, and Alabama). The Using Quality Parenting to Address Health arm utilizes a CBPR approach to identify community-prioritized health inequity conditions or specific diseases for children that could be addressed through quality parenting. The R24 planning project adapted the CCB model employed by the MSM PRC to prepare, plan, and develop quality parenting as an intervention for addressing community-identified health inequities in early and middle childhood through the SSC parenting initiative.[16] The overall goal is to develop and pilot test a community-driven plan that will result in parent-led efforts to mitigate health inequities among vulnerable minority children and families of low SES.

The Mayor's Healthy Communities Initiative

The Healthy Communities initiative, launched through MSM's Community Voices program in 2017, mobilizes and engages mayors, county officials, other elected officials, and their teams by enhancing their health leadership skills, providing community health resources, and motivating leaders to influence policies and implement health projects that will eliminate health disparities.[28] This program provides an opportunity for in-depth engagement in exploring topics that will give participants concrete tools to enable effective engagement of multidisciplinary sectors and resources required to improve health and community well-being. The yearlong program begins with a weeklong (48 hours) in-person intensive training where participants' health leadership knowledge and skills are enhanced. The intensive training consists of a series of workshops featuring an active learning approach where participants apply principles of leadership, integrate the impact of the social determinants of health, and work to develop competencies that result in community mobilization for health.

The Community Health Leadership Program

The CHLP is designed "to close the gap between academic medicine or academic health centers and the communities of greatest need by connecting to people who are most affected by disparities.[29, 30] The goal is to identify, develop, and enhance community health leaders who are educated, motivated, and mobilized to lead community groups in changing health behavior, improving environmental health, and influencing policies to support community health. CHLP consists of a series of workshops/seminars that build or enhance participant knowledge, skills, and leadership in mobilizing community groups toward changing health behaviors, improving environmental health, and influencing policies to support the establishment of healthier communities. The courses are presented in a flexible, learner-centered format via the classroom, the internet, audio conferencing, field-based practice, and modular social media design such as Facebook or Twitter to support learning and social organization. The curriculum is conducted as a nonintensive, 12-week training; an intensive three-day format; or an executive one-week training.

Atlanta Clinical and Translational Science Institute and the Georgia Clinical and Translational Science Alliance

Since their inception, both the ACTSI (2007–2017) and the more recently funded Georgia CTSA (2017–22) CE programs have been designed to (1) increase the capacities of community partners and academic researchers to develop and extend research projects to better address community priorities and (2) facilitate community-engaged partnerships that advance population health. Platforms for trainings include lunch and learns, half-day sessions, or breakout sessions infused into a recurring community-engaged research forum attracting leaders and learners from across the state of Georgia and beyond. A frequently requested topic is grant writing, addressing the challenges for community leaders with strong relationships and fingers on the pulse of the community to package their wisdom and plans into competitive grant proposals. Topics for grant writing workshops include (1) components of federal and nonfederal grants, (2) development of goals and objectives, (3) local data access and utilization, (4) logic model development, (5) specific aims/research question development, (6) strategy development, (7) budget development, and (8) the fundamentals of community-academic partnerships and projects. Examples of other workshops designed to facilitate community-led or co-created research and related partnerships are as follows:

- Community-Engaged Research Partnerships: Success, Lessons Learned, and Reflections—Finding a Partner
- Using Big Data to Analyze Health Disparities
- Evaluation—Building the Evidence to Demonstrate Impacts and Outcomes
- How to Establish and Maintain 501(c)(3) Nonprofit Status
- Are You a Community or Academic Potential Researcher Seeking a Partner?

MSM Pipeline Programs

Conceived by MSM president, the Office for Educational Outreach and Health Careers (EOHC) was established in 2012. The Office for EOHC oversees and directs all pipeline programs at the institution providing science, technology, engineering, arts, and mathematics exposure and mentoring opportunities for students from elementary through post-undergraduate levels. The MSM mission specifically commits to increasing the diversity of the health care workforce, emphasizing primary care, and serving the underserved. MSM has over 15 pipeline programs focused on students from K–12 through post-baccalaureate, coordinated by a single office and reaching thousands of students annually. The office is fueled by a commitment to increasing the number of underrepresented persons in medicine, the health professions, and the scientific workforce. The EOHC pipeline programs enhance educational opportunities in STEAM disciplines, intensify exposure to cutting-edge biomedical and public health research, and provide preparation for successful application to and matriculation in schools emphasizing careers in the health professions (see table 6.1).

MSM has centralized its efforts toward providing STEAM training, mentoring, and exposure to students of Atlanta Public Schools (APS). APS is one of the largest districts in the United States, with 52,000 students across 88 schools. Over 1,000 students and parents have been mentored or trained through interventions and programs offered by the EOHC office. More recently, MSM and the Tuskegee Airmen Global Academy have collaborated to centralize efforts designed to advance the skills and capacities of students, teachers, and parents. MSM employees, alumni, and students provide on-site mentoring for grades 2–5. Mentors are trained through the Atlanta CARES Mentoring Network and cleared as APS volunteers. Consequently, MSM was honored with the APS 2016 and 2017 Washington Cluster Partner of the Year Awards, as well as the 2016 School-Based Partner of the Year Award.

Summary

The school's mission reflects a not-so-hidden curriculum of primary care, service to the underserved, and disparities reduction that permeates the regular curriculum. MSM is dedicated to expanding educational programs and sustaining the highest standards of teaching excellence and professional competence. But far beyond the training of enrolled students and residents, its community-engaged educational impact is deep and far-reaching. MSM emphasizes the leadership and promotion of CHWs as central leaders in research, education, clinical, and service teams based on their understanding of or lived experience as members of priority populations, with strengths, resilience, and resources that often equal or outweigh the health risk factors that are too frequently

Table 6.1 Morehouse School of Medicine Pipeline Programs

Name of pipeline program	Educational level	Description
MSM-Tuskegee Academic CONNECT	Elementary	This program is a partnership between Morehouse School of Medicine, Tuskegee Airmen Global Academy, Atlanta Public Schools, and Atlanta CARES. The employees of Morehouse School of Medicine provide one-on-one and group mentoring to the third- through fifth-grade students.
MSM STEAM Academy (grades 4–8)	Elementary and middle school	Children are engaged in activities designed to increase their love of STEAM while helping to improve critical thinking/problem-solving skills and creativity (2–6 weeks). Students are involved in challenging hands-on interactive exercises that are designed to make learning science and math fun. Curricular activities, including the arts, are an integrated program of study.
Community Health Worker Training Program	High school	Year-long training program that seeks to increase the number of trained HSYACHWs to engage family, peers, and community in strategies for better health and wellness.
MSM STEAM Academy	High school	This program introduces students to biomedical research and health careers. Participants in this summer experience will be immersed in scientific instrumentation and laboratory techniques, as well as participate in mini-courses and workshops on health equity, careers in the sciences and health professions, critical thinking, and career planning.
First Look Health TEAM	High school	A day dedicated to exploring the exciting world of health careers. Participants must be currently enrolled in science- and technology-based curricula and will have the opportunity to work with MSM students, residents, and faculty in a workshop setting.
Reach One Each One	High school	A collaboration of Grady Health System, Morehouse School of Medicine, and Emory School of Medicine, the program is designed to introduce and expose high-performing students from underrepresented backgrounds who are interested in pursuing medical careers to various specialties during an intensive 10-week course.
Atlanta Sickle Cell Summer Research Program	High school	Sponsored by the Excellence in Hemoglobinopathies Research Award from the National Heart, Lung, and Blood Institute of the National Institutes of Health, this summer program was designed to involve young people from groups underrepresented in health professions and biomedical sciences through cutting-edge scientific research conducted in an academic medical center and to cultivate a continued interest in research related to sickle cell disease.
Short-Term Research Experience for Underrepresented Persons	High school and undergraduate	Sponsored by the National Institutes of Health, this program provides hands-on summer research experience (8–10 weeks) for high school and undergraduate students interested in exploring research careers.
Academically Prepared for Excellence	Undergraduate/ graduate students	The 10-week program identifies and recruits highly motivated, economically or educationally disadvantaged students, and those students who are underrepresented in medicine, who have a demonstrated potential and ability to pursue a career in medicine. The program is especially designed for students who have completed a bachelor's degree and may not have been successful on previous attempts to enter medical school.

used to characterize them. MSM, as a national and global CE pillar, has positioned itself as a well-recognized leader in training and technical assistance for researchers, practitioners, policy makers, and neighborhood residents, across the life course, to build, sustain, and assess community health partnerships. The examples described in this chapter are by no means exhaustive but serve to demonstrate the ways in which MSM strategically develops and promotes well-equipped CE leaders employing strategies that catalyze population health transformation.

References

1. "Community Health Workers." American Public Health Association. https://www.apha.org/apha-communities/member-sections/community-health-workers.

2. Blumenthal, D. S., J. Sung, R. Coates, J. Williams, and J. Liff. 1995. "Recruitment and Retention of Subjects for a Longitudinal Cancer Prevention Study in an Inner-City Black Community." *Health Services Research* 30 (1 pt. 2): 197–205.

3. "Choice Neighborhoods—Transforming Housing, Neighborhoods and People." Choice Atlanta. http://cnatlanta.org/about.php.

4. Pemu, Priscilla E., Alexander Q. Quarshie, R. Josiah-Willock, Folake O. Ojutalayo, Ernest Alema-Mensah, and Elizabeth O. Ofili. 2011. "Socio-demographic Psychosocial and Clinical Characteristics of Participants in e-HealthyStrides©: An Interactive ehealth Program to Improve Diabetes Self-Management Skills." *Journal of Health Care for the Poor and Underserved* 22 (4 Suppl.): 146–64. doi:10.1353/hpu.2011.0162.

5. Ofili, Elizabeth O., Priscilla E. Pemu, Alexander Quarshie, Ernest Alema Mensah, Latrice Rollins, Folake Ojutalayo, Atuarra McCaslin, and Bethany Saint Clair. 2018. "DEMOCRATIZING DISCOVERY HEALTH WITH N=Me." *Transactions of the American Clinical and Climatological Association* 129:215–34.

6. "Health360x." Morehouse School of Medicine. http://www.health360x.com/.

7. Smith, Selina A., and Daniel S. Blumenthal. 2012. "Community Health Workers Support Community-Based Participatory Research Ethics: Lessons Learned along the Research-to-Practice-to-Community Continuum." *Journal of Health Care for the Poor and Underserved* 23 (4 Suppl.): 77–87.

8. Blumenthal, D. S., S. A. Smith, C. D. Majett, and E. Alema-Mensah. 2010. "A Trial of Three Interventions to Promote Colorectal Cancer Screening in African Americans." *Cancer* 116 (4): 922–29.

9. Smith, S. A., L. Johnson, D. Wesley, K. B. Turner, G. McCray, J. Sheats, and D. Blumenthal. 2012. "Translation to Practice of an Intervention to Promote Colorectal Cancer Screening among African Americans." *Clinical and Translational Science* 5 (5): 412–15.

10. Smith, S. A., and D. S. Blumenthal. 2013. "Efficacy to Effectiveness Transition of an Educational Program to Increase Colorectal Cancer Screening (EPICS): Study Protocol of a Cluster Randomized Controlled Trial." *Implementation Science* 8:86.

11. Daniels, Elvan C., Barbara D. Powe, Toye Metoyer, Gail McCray, Peter Baltrus, and George S. Rust. 2012. "Increasing Knowledge of Cardiovascular Risk

Factors among African Americans by Use of Community Health Workers: The ABCD Community Intervention Pilot Project." *Journal of the National Medical Association* 104 (3–4): 179–85.

12. Josiah Willock, Robina, Robert M. Mayberry, Fengxia Yan, and Pamela Daniels. 2015. "Peer Training of Community Health Workers to Improve Heart Health among African American Women." *Health Promotion Practice* 16 (1): 63–71. doi:10.1177/1524839914535775.

13. Bolar, Cassandra L., Natalie Hernandez, Tabia Henry Akintobi, Calvin McAllister, Aneeqah S. Ferguson, Latrice Rollins, Glenda Wrenn, Martha Okafor, David Collins, and Thomas Clem. 2016. "Context Matters: A Community-Based Study of Urban Minority Parents' Views on Child Health." *Journal of the Georgia Public Health Association* 5 (3): 212–19.

14. Okafor, Martha, Daniel F. Sarpong, Aneeqah Ferguson, and David Satcher. 2013. "Improving Health Outcomes of Children through Effective Parenting: Model and Methods." *International Journal of Environmental Research and Public Health* 11 (1): 296–311. doi:10.3390/ijerph110100296.

15. Henry Akintobi, T., et al. 2017. "Advancing Community-Based Participatory Research from Start to Finish: A Community Engagement Model to Support a Center of Excellence on Health Disparities." American Public Health Association Annual Meeting & Expo, Atlanta, GA.

16. Akintobi, T. H., et al. 2018. "Processes and Outcomes of a Community-Based Participatory Research-Driven Health Needs Assessment: A Tool for Moving Health Disparity Reporting to Evidence-Based Action." *Progress in Community Health Partnerships: Research, Education, and Action* 12 (1S): 139–47.

17. Akintobi, T. H., et al. 2016. "Applying a Community-Based Participatory Research Approach to Address Determinants of Cardiovascular Disease and Diabetes Mellitus in an Urban Setting." In *Handbook of Community-Based Participatory Research*, ed. S. Coughlin, S. Smith, and M. Fernandez, 131–54. New York: Oxford University Press.

18. Rollins, L., T. Akintobi, A. Hermstad, D. Cooper, L. Goodin, J. Beane, S. Spivey, A. Riedesel, L. Taylor, and R. Lyn. 2017. "Community-Based Approaches to Reduce Chronic Disease Disparities in Georgia." *Journal of the Georgia Public Health Association* 6 (4): 402–10.

19. Quarells, R., W. Thompson, E. Yancey, L. Rollins, T. H. Akintobi, and S. Genzyme. 2019. *Community Engagement and Health Disparities in Clinical and Translational Research Course: A Joint Academic Institution Approach*. Washington, DC: Association for Clinical and Translational Science Annual Meeting.

20. Weiner, Stacy. 2018. "Little-Known Health Workers, Coming Soon to a Hospital Near You." *AAMC News*, December 4, 2018.

21. Morehouse School of Medicine—Digital Learning. HSCHW Promo 2018, May 25, 2018. https://youtu.be/MB22veMGTCk.

22. Blumenthal, D., R. DiClemente, R. Braithwaite, and S. Smith, eds. 2013. *Community-Based Participatory Health Research: Issues, Methods, and Translation to Practice*. 2nd ed. New York: Springer.

23. Blumenthal, D. S., and R. J. DiClemente. 2004. *Community-Based Health Research: Issues and Methods*. New York: Springer.

24. "Community Health Advanced by Medical Practice Superstars Transformational Leadership Fellowship." Morehouse School of Medicine. https://www.msm.edu/Education/champs/index.php.

25. "HEAL Clinic—Community Service Opportunities." Morehouse School of Medicine. http://www.msm.edu/Current_Students/currentStudents_commservice.php.

26. Akintobi, T. H., et al. 2016. "Flipping the Script: Increasing Urban Minority Residents' Capacities to Engage as Equal or Senior Partners in Behavioral and Clinical Research." American Public Health Association 144th Annual Conference, Denver, CO.

27. "Satcher Health Leadership Institute." http://satcherinstitute.org/.

28. "NCCDPHP: Community Health." Centers for Disease Control and Prevention. https://www.cdc.gov/nccdphp/dch/programs/healthycommunitiesprogram/communities/overallmap.htm.

29. Hairston-Blanks, Starla. 2016. "Healthy Communities Initiative." Satcher Health Leadership Institute. http://satcherinstitute.org/healthy-communities-initiative/.

30. Hairston-Blanks, Starla. 2016. "Community Health Leadership Program." http://satcherinstitute.org/community-health-leadership-program/.

SEVEN

The Medical School of Tomorrow

To UNDERSTAND the characteristics of the Medical School of Tomorrow, we need to start with the Medical School of Yesterday. This chapter will begin by examining the medical education reforms that occurred in the early twentieth century and the baseline they established for the medical education changes that followed. There is a trajectory to these changes, and by extrapolating this trajectory into the next few decades, we may be able to envision what medical education will look like in the middle of the twenty-first century. Morehouse School of Medicine (MSM) is, in many ways, on the leading edge of this trajectory. A review of some aspects of the MSM experience may assist with this prognostication. We must acknowledge that in the first part of the twenty-first century there exists much churning of ideas and initiatives. While the Morehouse experience does not fully represent the breadth of change, it is a significant player in the emerging changes.

The Flexner Report and Its Impact

Prior to the twentieth century, medical education was mostly unregulated and far from standardized. The reality was a "wild west" of teaching institutions that ranged from university-based programs to proprietary schools owned by individual physicians whose own training might have been suspect. At the proprietary schools, basic science might or might not be taught, and prerequisite education was whatever the school's owner thought necessary. Some of the schools essentially offered apprenticeships.

In the early part of the twentieth century, the American Medical Association (AMA) began to take a dim view of this state of affairs. In 1904, it created its Council on Medical Education, consisting of five professors of medicine from major universities. The council was charged with taking action to improve and standardize medical education in the United States. It began by recommending a minimum period of education for physicians of four years of high school, four years of medical school, and passage of a licensing examination; ideally, there would be five years of medical school, including a year of basic sciences, and a sixth year consisting of a hospital internship.[1] The AMA subsequently investigated and rated medical schools according to whether they met these standards, as well as standards of curriculum, faculty, facilities, admission requirements, and graduates' rates of passage of state licensing examinations. It identified 82 schools of which they fully approved (Class A), 46 that needed improvement (Class B), and 32 that were considered irredeemable (Class C).[1]

However, the AMA never released the results of this study. Instead, in 1908 it asked the Carnegie Foundation for the Advancement of Teaching to investigate and evaluate American medical education. To conduct this study, the commission chose Abraham Flexner, a young educator with a bachelor's degree from Johns Hopkins University. Mr. Flexner had no medical or health science–related background but had previously published a critique of American higher education entitled *The American College: A Criticism.* Ironically, he was the owner of a proprietary college in Louisville, Kentucky.

Apparently, Flexner undertook this effort virtually single-handedly, unlike more recent deliberative bodies that have been charged with making recommendations on medical education, such as the Graduate Medical Education National Advisory Committee (1981)[2] or the Council on Graduate Medical Education (1990, and subsequent reports).[3] These and other bodies composed a sizable team of experts, assisted by a staff. Flexner, however, personally visited all 155 American and

Canadian medical schools (there were only two medical schools in Canada at the time).

Flexner's report was published in 1910. It was entitled *Medical Education in the United States and Canada: A Report to the Carnegie Foundation for the Advancement of Teaching*.[4] This report is more generally known as simply the "Flexner Report" (or, by the cognoscenti, as "Bulletin Number Four") and was as scathing as one might have imagined, given the state of medical education in the first decade of the twentieth century. Flexner recommended that the number of medical schools be reduced to 31, generally conforming to the "Class A" schools identified by the AMA. He also made the following recommendations:[5]

- Increase the prerequisites to enter medical training: a high school degree, plus at least two years of college, primarily focused on basic science.
- Train physicians to practice in a scientific manner and engage medical faculty in research.
- Give medical schools control of clinical instruction in hospitals.
- Medical schools should be part of a university.
- Strengthen state regulation of medical licensure.
- The medical curriculum should consist of two years of basic science plus two years of hospital-based clinical work.

Flexner is often credited with establishing the curricular model of two years of basic science followed by two clinical years. However, this is the model that had been recommended by the AMA's Council on Medical Education in 1904 and was the model used by the Johns Hopkins University School of Medicine, which was considered by Flexner to be the ideal medical school. Even today, schools designing curricula that deviate from this model generally state that they are departing from the Flexnerian model. Similarly, Flexner is usually given credit for launching the reforms in medical education that followed his report. In reality, the report might more accurately be viewed as providing stimulus to reforms that had already begun. For instance, the number of medical schools had dropped from a high point of 162 in 1906 to 131 in 1910, the year the Flexner Report was published.[1]

Flexner's famous document also led to, or supported, changes that might be viewed with disfavor today. For instance, five of the seven medical schools that admitted Black students closed. The two survivors were Howard University School of Medicine and Meharry Medical College. Flexner viewed the role of the Black physician as one "limited to his own race." The focus of these physicians, he argued, should be on controlling infectious diseases among Blacks, thus preventing their spread to Whites.[6] Needless to say, discrimination against Blacks at the predominantly White schools of medicine existed at the time of Flexner and persisted—perhaps to the present day.

As the number of young people admitted to medical school was reduced as a result of Flexner-era reforms, the number of women admitted decreased, disproportionately. Flexner thought that the declining number of women medical students reflected diminishing demand for their services or diminishing interest in the profession on the part of women. However, many medical college administrators argued that women physicians would cease to practice after marriage and that discrimination against their admission to medical school was therefore justified. Quotas that limited women to about 5 percent of medical school classes existed at least until the 1970s, except during wartime.[7]

The Decades after Flexner

In the 25 years after the publication of the Flexner Report, over half of US medical schools closed. By 1935, only 66 schools were operating.[8] With the loss of so many schools, the number of practicing physicians began to dwindle, and as the population grew, the physician-to-population ratio was markedly reduced. There were calls for increasing class sizes and creating new medical schools, but the medical establishment resisted. In 1934, the incoming president of the AMA called for the *closure* of half the schools,[9] and the AMA expressed opposition to enlarging class sizes. By the 1960s, however, the doctor shortage became undeniable, and the federal government made funds available to create new medical schools. Between 1965 and 1980, with the aid of these funds, the number of schools grew from 88 to 126, and the annual number of graduates rose from 7,409 to 15,135.[10] MSM was one of those schools.

The official founding year of MSM was 1975—the year that the school's first dean, Dr. Louis W. Sullivan, took up his position. The first class of 24 students was admitted in 1979. At that time, it was not actually a school, but rather the Medical Education Program at Morehouse College. In 1981, the planned separation of Morehouse College and MSM took place. Morehouse College continues as a historically Black four-year liberal arts college for men. Both, however, are part of the geographically contiguous Atlanta University Center, along with Spelman College (a four-year liberal arts college for women), Clark Atlanta University, Morris Brown College, and the Interdenominational Theological Center.

The year 1981 was also the year in which MSM admitted the first students who would spend all four years of their medical education at the school and receive a MSM diploma. Until then, MSM offered only the first two years of medical school—the basic science years—and all the students then had to transfer to other, four-year schools to complete their degree. Several schools had agreed to accept MSM students who completed their first two years satisfactorily and passed the national "Board Exam" that is given at the end of the second year of medical school.

From a national medical education perspective, the most important event of 1981 was the publication of the Report of the Graduate Medical Education National Advisory Committee, or GMENAC (commonly pronounced "Geminack").[2] This committee was chartered by the Secretary of the Department of Health, Education, and Welfare (now the US Department of Health and Human Services) "to analyze the distribution of specialties among physicians and residents and to evaluate alternative approaches to ensure an appropriate balance." It was directed to "make recommendations to the Secretary on overall strategies on the present and future supply and requirements of physicians by specialty ... ; (and) translation of physician requirements into a range of types and numbers of graduate training opportunities needed to approach a more desirable distribution of physician services."[11]

Using complex modeling strategies, the committee concluded that by 1990 there would be an excess of about 70,000 physicians overall, and major surpluses in some specialties, for instance, cardiology (7,750), general surgery (nearly 10,000), and obstetrics-gynecology (over 10,000). Other specialties—notably those in primary care—would be in near balance, and some, such as emergency medicine and preventive medicine, would be in short supply.[12] Among other recommendations, the committee stated that the number of minorities in medicine should be increased.

The committee recommended a 10 percent decrease in the number of medical students relative to the 1978–79 level, a recommendation that was not met with joy by the medical education establishment. Few schools actually reduced their class sizes, but there was widespread concern that a "doctor glut" was in the offing.

By the early 2000s, the pendulum was beginning to swing in the other direction. Newer physician manpower analyses demonstrated an incipient doctor *shortage*. An early proponent of this perspective was Dr. Richard Cooper, who in 2002 predicted a shortage of physicians in general,[13] and in particular a shortage of specialists.[14] This view was more readily accepted by medical schools and by universities that longed to have medical schools. The Association of American Medical Colleges adopted models that progressively showed larger and larger deficits; in 2018 the projected physician shortage by 2030 had reached as many as 120,000 physicians.[15]

How did expert analyses reach such disparate conclusions? The GMENAC analysis used a *need-based* planning model that asked, "How many physicians will be needed?" Given, for instance, the number of individuals with heart disease at the time of the study and in the future, how many primary care physicians and cardiologists would be needed to care for them? By contrast, the later analyses used a *demand-based* model: given a market-based health care delivery system that sells as much health care as people with means (cash and insurance) wish to buy, how many physicians will be required to meet that demand?

With the projections now inverted, a medical school boom ensued. By 2018, there were 141 accredited MD-granting institutions and 31 accredited DO (doctor of osteopathy) granting institutions in the United States. These were in addition to the 31 "offshore" medical schools in the Caribbean region. These are for-profit schools that cater to Americans who are unable to gain admission to US medical schools.

Hence, we are able to see how the activities of the twentieth century have established the trajectory of medical education in the twenty-first century. Flexner and the regulatory bodies that he influenced created a new focus on quality in medical education, a focus that continues to grow stronger, as we shall see in the pages that follow. "Quality" in this sense does not just mean better lectures (in fact, lectures are becoming progressively less important) but also includes the environment in which the education takes place, the tools that are used, and the extent to which educational opportunities are being extended to students who were previously denied them. It also includes the application of the social justice principles described in chapter 2.

In addition, Flexner set in motion a pendulum-like process that initially led to a reduction in the number of medical schools and medical students, then an increase starting in the 1960s, then a decrease (or at least a leveling off) in the 1970s, and now, starting in the 2000s, a renewed increase.

Going forward, however, the number of practicing physicians may be limited by the number of available residency positions. Most US residency programs are supported by Medicare, and there is reluctance on the part of the US Congress to grow Medicare by increasing expenditures for resident training (rather than actual medical care). While there has been some growth in residency positions, it has been small compared to the growth in US medical graduates. Hence, the competition for desirable residency slots has become more intense. Residency programs favor graduates from US schools, so graduates of offshore and foreign schools are likely to struggle even more than they currently do to find residency positions.

Hence, we come to one characteristic of *the Medical School of Tomorrow: it will need to prepare its students to be ever more competitive in the residency marketplace.* Competition is already hyperintense for positions in some subspecialties, such as dermatology, radiology,

How Did Morehouse Get Started?

It was a time of turmoil in medical education. The first steps toward the creation of Morehouse School of Medicine took place in 1968, but the official year of founding was 1975. It was a time of medical school expansion: conventional wisdom and learned reports described a physician shortage, and many new medical schools were coming on line. Federal funds to support this growth were plentiful.

But the field was beginning to reverse. President Richard M. Nixon (1968–74) recognized that health care costs were mounting, and more medical schools and more doctors would mean more expense. The 1981 GMENAC Report completed the reversal: according to the report, the United States was not facing a doctor shortage, but rather a doctor surplus. This occurred just as MSM was seeking funds from the state of Georgia to remain sustainable. State legislators were pushing back.

The MSM argument was that, notwithstanding national data regarding the physician workforce, there was a clear shortage of Black doctors in the nation at large and, specifically, in Georgia. For instance, there were 795 White Georgians for every White doctor in the state but 13,810 Black Georgians for every Black doctor.

Still, prospects for support from the mostly White and rural legislature were not great. However, at virtually the same time, a new medical school was being developed at Mercer University, a predominantly White Baptist school located in Macon, Georgia. Its mission was to graduate primary care physicians for rural Georgia. In the end, there was a trade-off: White rural legislators who favored Mercer and Black Atlanta legislators who favored Morehouse agreed to support both schools.

References
1. Gasman, M. 2012. *The Morehouse Mystique*. Baltimore: Johns Hopkins University Press.

plastic surgery, orthopedics, and ophthalmology. Students pursuing these positions may interview with 20 or more programs across the country in an attempt to gain acceptance into one.

MSM has some advantages in this arena. First, it focuses on preparing students for primary care careers, and residencies in these fields—family medicine, general pediatrics, and general internal medicine—are among the least competitive. Second, many residency programs, wishing to increase the diversity of their resident corps, try to recruit well-qualified underrepresented minorities. This description fits most MSM graduates.

New Developments: Heading for Tomorrow

In this section, we will examine newer developments in medical education and consider the ways in which these developments may progress in the future, leading to the "Medical School of Tomorrow." Morehouse is a leader in some of these areas; in others, not.

Simulation

Computer models and simulations are serving as "teaching material," partially replacing humans. In the anatomy lab, for instance, computerized models of humans allow students to peel back layers of skin and muscle by touching a life-sized screen. In some medical schools in the United Kingdom and Australia, this type of simulation has completely replaced cadaver dissection. In the United States it remains supplemental. Comparisons of anatomy learned entirely by simulation versus anatomy learned by cadaver dissection appear to give an edge to the cadaver method,[16, 17] although the magnitude of the advantage is not clear.[18]

Computerized simulators perform a variety of functions previously available only through patient contact. One can examine a life-sized dummy and auscultate heart murmurs, breath sounds, or bowel sounds. The dummy, or another simulation model, can be used to practice intubation, endoscopy, or other procedures.

"Standardized patients" could also be considered a type of simulation, although this approach utilizes humans. Standardized patients are individuals who are trained to simulate subjective and objective findings of diseases and conditions. Their use in medical education grew widely in the 1990s and continues today.[19] Students perform histories and physical examinations on the standardized patients and then receive feedback on their skills. Standardized patients are also used in examinations of students. At MSM, students perform histories and physicals on standardized patients in exam rooms equipped with video cameras. Faculty in a remote room observe the students on monitors, critique their performance, and make recommendations for improvements.

In the Medical School of Tomorrow, there will be more simulations, and they will be ever more realistic. A humanoid robot, using artificial intelligence, will give a complete history in response to the student's questions, and the student will be able to perform a complete physical examination. According to the requirements of the day's lesson, the spleen or the liver could be enlarged, an inguinal hernia could be palpated, or any type of rash could develop. In view of the speed with which technology has developed during the past couple of decades, if the reader of this book has not acquired the book within a year or two of publication, it is likely that this robot and other remarkable simulations will already be available.

Ultimately, clinical learning takes place on real patients, but the patients are spared some of the students' initial efforts if the students have practiced first through simulations. Simulations will become more and more realistic in the future, but learning is a lifelong process that, necessarily, involves real patients.

CASE STUDY: The Medical School of the Distant Future

In *Star Trek*, the science fiction TV series of the 1960s that later gave birth to several movies, Dr. Leonard McCoy is the chief medical officer for the starship *Enterprise*, having been posted in the year 2266. He has neither stethoscope nor reflex hammer but instead uses a tricorder, a handheld scanner that, when passed over the body of an ill individual, provides an instant diagnosis and instructions for treating the ailment. It even works on aliens from other planets.

There doesn't seem to be any special skill or training needed to operate the tricorder, which suggests that in the twenty-third century the course of study to become a physician will be very short indeed.

The Internet

In many ways, the internet has revolutionized education. Entire courses can now be taken online, and the student need never leave home. Answers to questions can be gathered with the click of a mouse. Students need not attend lectures but can view video-recorded lectures at any time and place. Courses, lectures, journals, and other written materials can be offered to people in developing countries who would not otherwise have access to any of these things. At MSM, students can access much educational material online, but the option to "never leave home" is not offered.

Research has shown that internet-based education is as effective as traditional methods, although some students may learn better than others through this approach.[20] *In the Medical School of Tomorrow, internet-based education will play a major role.*

Curriculum Reform

Flexner's prescribed medical school curriculum—two years of basic science followed by two years of clinical education in the hospital—persisted, unchanged, in "cookie-cutter" fashion at nearly every medical school, at least until the 1980s. The basic science years consisted of courses in anatomy, histology, physiology, and biochemistry in the first year and pathology, pharmacology, and microbiology in the second year. Schools considered pioneers of change began by teaching basic science in a "systems-oriented" fashion. That is, the basic science of the cardiovascular system was considered in one module, that of the nervous system in another, and so forth. However, this sort of change mostly amounted to rearranging the sequence of lectures, rather than a fundamental change in educational approach.

The early signs of more radical change came in the 1980s, when curricula featuring problem-based teaching and learning were introduced at McMaster University in Canada, as well as at schools in the Netherlands and Australia. The first adopters in the United States were Southern Illinois University, Michigan State University, and the University of

New Mexico. Howard Barrows, who had pioneered the use of standardized patients as early as 1968,[21] was its chief proponent.[22]

In problem-based teaching and learning, students rarely or never sit at lectures. Rather, to learn basic science, they are presented with descriptions of clinical problems and, working in small groups, turn to books, simulations, online information, and consultations with professors to solve the problems. In so doing, they learn basic science and generally enjoy the process more than do the students who attend lectures.

These early curriculum reform initiatives led to a wave of innovations that veered substantially from the Flexnerian model. Additional schools adopted some version of problem-based teaching, sometimes in combination with more traditional methods. Patient contact was introduced in the first year of medical school. Significant clinical teaching was done in the outpatient clinic. Systems-oriented integrated basic science curricula became widespread. Interprofessional components were introduced, so that medical students learned alongside students of nursing, pharmacy, and other health professions.[23] Required research experiences were added. Longitudinal integrated clerkships that simulate a family practice replaced block clerkships.[24] Three-year programs were introduced, fell,[25] and then rose again.[26] Dual-degree programs in which students enrolled in an MD program simultaneously pursue a master's degree or a PhD are widespread (and some have been in place at least since the 1960s). More sophisticated educational concepts are being employed, and medical educators are placing an emphasis on "educators," rather than assuming that any skilled clinician is also an excellent teacher. Faculty members with advanced degrees in education are commonplace. Research on improved educational methodology is widely published. Specialized journals (*Academic Medicine*, *Medical Teacher*, *Education for Health*, and others) are largely dedicated to publishing research on educational methodology.

MSM has partaken of some items on this menu of change, but not all. For instance, the school now employs a systems-oriented integrated basic science curriculum. First-year students have had patient contact, mostly in primary care settings, since the school was established. They also have extensive community contact through the community health course, which is taught in small groups in the community. Substantial parts of the clinical curriculum take place in outpatient settings, often in community locations. The school offers dual MD-MPH and MD-PhD degrees. On the other hand, interprofessional education is difficult to implement, since MSM is a free-standing medical school, rather than part of a university that includes schools of nursing, pharmacy, and so on.

When it comes to medical education, the genie is out of the lamp. *The traditional Flexnerian model has been greatly disrupted and in the Medical School of Tomorrow will become even more disrupted.*

Kinder, Gentler Teaching

Traditionally, medical education has been considered a grueling experience, with domineering professors who enjoy humiliating students on rounds if they fall short of expectations. Abuse of students is common, is most often verbal, and includes sexual harassment. This is not part of the Flexnerian model, but rather a mode of teaching and an exploitation of power differentials passed on from one generation of professors of medicine to the next. The phenomenon was recognized and written about decades ago.[27] In more recent times, it has come to be recognized as counterproductive and downright destructive at its worst, possibly even leading to student suicide attempts. Unsurprisingly, minorities report the most incidents of mistreatment.[28] Policies and programs to prevent student abuse have been adopted at many medical schools, with little improvement.[29, 30]

A sympathetic approach to teaching has been emphasized at MSM, and faculty members consistently get positive ratings and informal praise from students regarding their supportive educational style. This is more the result of the school's educational ethic and atmosphere than a formal articulated policy (although abuse of students is indeed contrary to policy). This is necessarily where the Medical School of Tomorrow is headed. Too much attention has been focused on student abuse for it to continue unabated. While incidents will certainly still occur, students are now encouraged to report abuse, and schools have recognized the need to sensitize faculty and residents.

Hence, *the Medical School of Tomorrow will feature a more congenial learning environment than has been the case in the past and will not tolerate sexual harassment of students.*

Racial discrimination may be more difficult to eliminate, since much of it is subtle and due to "implicit racism"—the tendency to discriminate even among individuals who think they are treating everybody equally. All educational institutions dislike the idea that faculty or admissions committees may be discriminating against students of color, but many institutions have difficulty accepting the fact that such discrimination is taking place.

Hence, it is not clear that racial discrimination will ever be eliminated, but *the Medical School of Tomorrow will have programs in place to help prevent discrimination and will have feedback mechanisms to address it when it occurs.*

Eliminating Abuse and Discrimination in the Faculty

Abusive treatment is not limited to faculty abuse of students. Sexual harassment of junior faculty by those more senior is now recognized, and, belatedly, steps are being taken at many medical schools to eliminate it.[31]

Notice has also been taken of the failure of women to advance up the academic ladder in comparison to men at medical schools.[32] Women constitute about one-fifth of full-time faculty, but deanships, department chair positions, and full professorships go disproportionately to men. While this state of affairs has been exposed in recent years, it is not clear that adequate steps are being taken to rectify the situation. Moreover, the fact that Hispanic and African American medical school faculty (especially the latter) are less likely than White faculty to be promoted has been well documented.[33]

The Medical School of Tomorrow will have programs and processes to assist women and minorities to advance through the academic ranks and to ensure that they are not held back by discrimination. Sexual harassment of faculty will not be tolerated.

The Beyond Flexner Modalities and the Medical School of Tomorrow

In chapter 2, we examined the performance of MSM with respect to each of the modalities used in the Beyond Flexner study. Here, we project how the Medical School of Tomorrow (including MSM) will perform.

Mission

As pointed out in chapter 2, most medical school mission statements are vague and general. But since the growth period for medical schools in the 1960s and 1970s, numerous reports have emerged that point out the need for more primary care physicians, the need for more physicians in underserved communities, and the shortage of minority physicians. The MSM mission statement specifically addresses these needs (see chapter 2). Our expectation is that the Medical School of Tomorrow will follow suit. Medical schools established since 2000 have tended to respond to these issues and have created mission and vision statements that are more specific in this regard. For instance, the vision statement of the Quinnipiac University (CT) Netter School of Medicine (established in 2010) states that the school "will be a model for educating *diverse*, patient-centered physicians who are partners and leaders in an *inter-professional primary care* workforce responsive to *health care needs in the communities they serve*." The lengthy mission statement of the University of Houston School of Medicine (founded in 2018) refers specifically to primary care, diversity, and meeting the needs of "urban and rural areas of Texas that face significant doctor shortages." Not all new medical schools have mission statements that refer clearly to national, state, or local needs, however. For instance, the mission statement of the California University of Science and Medicine (founded in 2015) states that the school's mission is "to improve healthcare by training exceptional future physicians to advance the art and science of medicine through innovative medical education, research, and compassionate health care delivery." In general, though, it seems that *the Med-*

ical School of Tomorrow will be mission driven to respond to the most pressing needs of the country.

Pipeline

Building a "pipeline" to help underrepresented minorities qualify for medical school and develop an interest in a medical career is imperative to increasing diversity in medical education. It is an essential element at MSM. Without a pipeline to expand the minority applicant pool, medical schools that attempt to increase the diversity of their student body simply compete with each other and with programs in law, engineering, and so on, for the most qualified minorities. MSM has over 15 pipeline programs, including both summer and academic-year programs. Some of these reach elementary school students, while others reach high school and college students. Some involve laboratory research, while others are community based. Some are grant supported, while others are supported by the school.

At the national level, the Area Health Education Centers (AHEC) program, supported by both federal and state funds, builds pipelines at many of the nation's medical schools.[34] The MSM AHEC program was initiated shortly after the school was established; since 2016 it has participated in the Georgia Statewide AHEC Network. Outside of AHEC, it appears that there are few pipeline programs at schools of medicine (schools of nursing and dentistry may do better). Some of the more established programs are at the University of Washington,[35] the University of Illinois at Chicago,[36] Stanford University,[37] and the Ohio University College of Osteopathic Medicine.[38] Despite the long history of AHEC (since 1972) and the scattering of other programs, African Americans, Hispanics, and Native Americans remain badly underrepresented in US medical schools. *The Medical School of Tomorrow will develop stronger pipeline programs when it is serious about addressing this issue.*

Admissions

Many medical schools have attempted to increase minority enrollment through one or another form of "affirmative action" in admissions, but Supreme Court rulings and legislation in some states have limited the extent to which race and ethnicity can be used in admission decisions.[39] Schools may still generally use a "holistic" admissions process that takes into consideration many factors, including race and ethnicity. These may include, for instance, status as a first-generation college student, educational and socioeconomic status, geographic location, past experiences with minority and underserved populations, community service, and social capital. However, as this chapter is being written, the composition of the US Supreme Court is changing. The matter of admission to medical school and/or other institutions of higher learning is likely to come before the court again, and past rulings may be modified or overturned. *The Medical School of Tomorrow will attempt to admit a diverse class every year but will have to develop new strategies to do so.*[40]

Curriculum

The matter of overall curriculum reform was detailed earlier in this chapter. In the context of the "Beyond Flexner" modalities, it must be mentioned that many medical schools have introduced courses, clerkships, or experiences in minority health, health disparities, community health, and related topics, and some of these are quite creative. Social determinants—things like education, income, employment, neighborhood environment, powerlessness, and racism—are now recognized as the most important drivers of health status,[41] and they must be taught about in medical school.

Many courses in community health are still limited to lectures, or lectures plus a bus ride through some low-income communities. But increasingly, schools are developing courses and programs that provide students with hands-on service learning community experiences, sometimes under the banner of public health.[42] The MSM course and related programs, described in other chapters in this book, were among the first.

It should be noted that some schools in other countries have been lead-ers in this area.[43, 44] *Offering or (preferably) requiring community-based service learning experiences has become something of a movement. It is certain to be a feature of the Medical School of Tomorrow.*

Location of Clinical Experience

In 1961, Kerr White and colleagues, in what would become a classic paper, pointed out that about .4 percent of adults consulting a physi-cian for an illness were admitted to a university teaching hospital,[45] but that is where medical students received nearly all of their clinical edu-cation, as Flexner recommended. White updated the model in 1972,[46] and Green et al. did so again in 2001;[47] the findings were essentially the same. Despite this, it is only in relatively recent years that signifi-cant portions of clinical clerkships have been moved to the outpatient setting and, even more recently, that community practices have begun to serve as educational sites. Some schools now have tracks in which students receive major portions of their education in rural or inner-city ambulatory clinical sites. The A.T. Still School of Osteopathic Medicine sends all of its students to community health centers in several locations throughout the United States.[48] A few schools have rural tracks—for instance, Jefferson Medical College in Philadelphia[49] and the University of Illinois at Rockford.[50]

In addition, many schools (including MSM) offer rural or inner-city clerkships, which may be mandatory or may be electives. Students see-ing patients in these settings may, however, learn no more about the surrounding communities than they would if they were in a specialty clinic at the medical center. Unless the clerkship (or the track) in-cludes features that get the student out of the exam room and into the community—for instance, house calls or community projects—the ex-perience will represent wasted potential.

It must be noted here that, in at least some locations, there is a grow-ing competition for clerkship opportunities in community medical practices. Students from the offshore schools in the Caribbean receive only their basic science education at the home campus. Their clinical training takes place in the United States, and they must find—and pay—medical practices that will take them in. But since there is reason to hope that educational experiences in underserved communities will motivate students to practice in similar communities when they complete their training, such experiences are becoming more common.

Relatedly, increasing numbers of medical (and other health science) students are seeking experiences in developing countries. For some, this represents merely a bit of adventure, but others are contemplating a career that partially includes or is primarily focused on "global health." At the same time, the United States is adopting policies and programs to promote control of infectious diseases abroad out of concern about their possible spread to the United States.

The Medical School of Tomorrow will offer tracks in underserved communities and community clerkships that are part of the core curriculum. These clerkships will include experiences in the community, outside of the office or clinic. Similarly, global health tracks will appear, and clinical experiences in developing countries will be commonplace.

Tuition Management

The average medical school debt of graduating students rose from $179,000 in 2009 to $190,000 in 2016. When undergraduate debt is included, the average educational debt was $207,000. The driver of this debt is tuition increases, which have been substantially greater than inflation. Table 7.1 indicates the rate at which tuition and fees have been rising.

As the cost of a medical education skyrockets, low-income applicants—many of whom are minorities and rural residents—are discouraged

Table 7.1 Average Tuition and Fees, US Medical Schools

Academic year	Public schools, resident	Public schools, nonresident	Private schools, nonresident
1996–97	9,779	21,582	24,002
2017–18[a]	19,887	60,141	52,237

Note: Data from the Association of American Medical Colleges.
[a] Includes health insurance.

from pursuing a medical career.[51] Graduates are driven toward high-paying but overstocked subspecialties and away from lower-salary but critically needed primary care fields. Schools seek funds for scholarships (mostly from donations), but clearly insufficient scholarship funds are available, as evidenced by the student debt figures. From the schools' perspective, high tuition and fees may reduce their competitiveness for the most outstanding applicants, as well as hinder efforts to diversify their student bodies. On the other hand, tuition money is "unrestricted" and therefore particularly attractive. Grants and many donations are earmarked for particular projects or programs, but unrestricted funds can be spent for anything, from needed equipment to redecorating the dean's office.

Some schools have taken important steps. New York University School of Medicine announced in 2018 that all students, current and future, would receive full-tuition scholarships. At the time, the school was three-quarters of the way toward raising the $600 million needed to fund the initiative. The Kaiser Permanente School of Medicine announced that it will be waiving tuition for its first five graduating classes. Thirteen schools created accelerated three-year curricula, thus saving students a year's worth of tuition and fees, along with offering other advantages associated with one less year of school.

MSM—which annually admits a class composed of about 80 percent underrepresented minorities—struggles to raise adequate scholarship funds. At most schools, wealthy alumni are a major source of scholarship donations, but as a relatively new school, and one whose alumni body is largely composed of primary care physicians, MSM has few truly wealthy alumni. Nonetheless, the school is able to offer some scholarship support to about half of its students, as well as a partial debt repayment award given to all students at graduation.

Nationally, there is much agreement—in principle at least—that the current situation is unsustainable. *The Medical School of Tomorrow must find a way to limit the cost of attendance.*

Mentoring

Mentoring is generally thought to be a good thing, and it takes many different forms. It can happen one-on-one or in a group; it can focus on academics, research, or life in general;[52] it can consist of second-year students mentoring first-year students ("peer-to-peer");[53] and it can be part of a program to assist members of a group (e.g., racial/ethnic minority, female, LGBTQ) who may experience unique pressures as medical students.[54]

Learning communities, a form of group mentoring, are now very popular at US medical schools.[55] These can incorporate many types of mentoring (e.g., peer-to-peer, academics, life in general). But learning communities do not replace more traditional one-on-one mentoring, which may be particularly helpful for, for instance, minority students at a predominantly White institution. As described in chapter 2, MSM made mentoring a special priority. To increase the number and effectiveness of mentors at the school, it has established a "Mentoring Academy." It also plays a lead role in the National Research Mentoring Network, a National Institutes of Health–funded consortium of schools working to increase the number of underrepresented minorities in the biomedical research workforce.

It must also be recognized that mentoring relationships can go wrong as a result of harassment, abandonment, or just poor mentor-mentee fit. Still, with mostly "soft" and anecdotal evidence to support its benefits, *mentoring is regarded as important at most medical schools and will remain so at the Medical School of Tomorrow.*

Research of Tomorrow

Research is not a Beyond Flexner modality but is nonetheless an essential function of medical schools. Medical schools secure major research funding from NIH and other federal agencies, as well as foundations and pharmaceutical companies, and conduct highly sophisticated research at both the basic science and clinical levels. Through the AAMC and other organizations, such as Research!America, the schools have lobbied successfully for frequent increases in NIH funding. From 1994 to 2018, this funding increased from about $10 billion per year to nearly $40 billion per year. Much of this was due to a doubling of NIH funding between 1998 and 2003.[56] Few federal agencies have done as well.

The vast majority of NIH funding has supported high-tech research focused on such scientific niches as genomics, proteomics, and "precision medicine." These fields hold much promise for improved treatments of disease, particularly cancer treatments. However, there has been increased recognition that discoveries at academic institutions—even relatively low-tech discoveries—often do not find their way into community medical practices and into communities. Several years are required for this dissemination to take place. It is often stated that an average of 17 years are required for a new discovery to enter widespread practice.[57] For instance, only about half of people with high blood pressure have their condition under control.[58] This is despite the fact that low-cost antihypertensive drugs have been available for far more than 17 years and that simple lifestyle modifications can reduce blood pressure.

This has given rise to "translational research": research into improved approaches to "translating" basic science discoveries into new clinical tests and therapies, and thence into widespread use in communities and medical practices. In the early part of the twenty-first century, NIH initiated a program of major Clinical and Translational Science Awards (CTSA) to promote translational research. These multimillion-dollar grants established "hubs" at major research universities, and, as is typically the case with NIH grants, the focus of the programs is on basic and high-tech clinical research. But "community engagement" is a component of the hubs, and it is apparent to some, at least, that these components are essential if the new discoveries—and even the old discoveries—are to benefit the majority of the US population. For instance, more effective ways must be found to reach more people with screening for colorectal cancer, with treatment for hypertension, and to improve diets and physical activity. At the Georgia Clinical and Translational Science Alliance—the name of the multi-institutional CTSA on which Emory University serves as the prime grantee—CE is a major component, and this component is led by MSM.

Most of that community-engaged translational research will be CBPR (and similar approaches), which helps ensure that research conducted in communities does not violate ethical principles. This is particularly important in conducting research focused on reducing racial and ethnic health disparities, since the echoes of the infamous Tuskegee Syphilis Study (and other unethical research projects) still resound in minority communities. MSM's leadership in CBPR is discussed in chapter 4.

At the Medical School of Tomorrow, translational research will compose an ever-larger component of the research portfolio, and an increasingly large proportion of the translational research will be CBPR.

Service of Tomorrow

Like research, service is not a Beyond Flexner modality but is an essential function of medical schools. Historically, this was composed of highly specialized clinical services, and this will certainly continue to be the case in the future. However, there are increasing numbers of for-profit competitors in this space; a notable example is Cancer Treatment Centers of America. In order to "feed" their high-tech services, medical schools have established, or bought, many primary care practices. But these practices have become important to the medical schools for another reason: they are needed as teaching sites as the schools' educational function has shifted in the direction of primary care. To the extent that US medical schools can conduct teaching activities in their own primary care clinics, there is that much less need to compete with offshore Caribbean schools for student placement in community practices. Moreover, as a larger proportion of the population gains health insurance through the Affordable Care Act ("Obamacare") and other future initiatives, establishing medical school–affiliated primary care practices in less affluent communities becomes more feasible. *The Medical School of Tomorrow will be increasingly invested in primary care sites in both urban and rural communities.*

But as pointed out elsewhere in this book, clinical services are not the only services that medical schools should offer. MSM has been a leader among medical schools in providing health promotion and disease prevention services in low-income and minority communities. These programs are consistent with the MSM mission, but unlike clinical services, they are not inherently profitable. One cannot charge communities a fee for these services, so they must be supported by grants, donations, or volunteerism.

As medical schools throughout the United States are becoming more community oriented, they are establishing similar programs and are using them to expose their students to communities. They are discovering, too, that these programs are good for public relations.

Summary

The Medical School of Tomorrow will employ ever more sophisticated technology, will have an evolving curriculum that utilizes what educators now know about adult learning, and will employ teachers who do not abuse their students. Racial, ethnic, and gender-based discrimination will be greatly reduced.

Importantly, medical schools of tomorrow will be more socially accountable. Their classes will be more diverse than the schools of today. Compared to the present, they will graduate a higher percentage of students who will pursue primary care careers, work in underserved communities, and represent an underrepresented minority group. The schools will be more engaged in the community. Their research will increasingly focus on the priority health problems of communities, be prevention oriented, be conducted in an ethical fashion, and be developed, implemented, and disseminated in partnership with the communities where the research is conducted. They will offer services that are more oriented to health promotion and disease prevention and are provided at the community level. To achieve these research and service outcomes, they will work more closely with schools of public health or will elevate their own public health programs. MSM will continue to represent one model of the Medical School of Tomorrow.

References

1. Starr, Paul. 1982. *The Social Transformation of American Medicine*. New York: Basic Books.

2. Graduate Medical Education National Advisory Committee. 1981. *Report of the Graduate Medical Education National Advisory Committee to the Secretary, Department of Health and Human Services*. Washington, DC: US Department of Health and Human Services.

3. Council on Graduate Medical Education. 1990. *COGME: First Report*. Washington, DC: US Department of Health and Human Services.

4. Flexner, A. 1910. *Medical Education in the United States and Canada: A Report to the Carnegie Foundation for the Advancement of Teaching*. Bulletin No. 4 of the Carnegie Foundation for the Advancement of Teaching. New York. http:// archive.carnegiefoundation.org/pdfs/elibrary/Carnegie_Flexner_Report.pdf.

5. Barzansky, Barbara, and Norman Gevitz. 1992. *Beyond Flexner: Medical Education in the Twentieth Century*. New York: Greenwood.

6. Sullivan, L. W., and I. S. Mittman. 2010. "The State of Diversity in the Health Professions a Century after Flexner." *Academic Medicine* 85 (2): 246–53.

7. Starr, Paul. 1982. *The Social Transformation of American Medicine*, 124. New York: Basic Books.

8. Hiatt, Mark D., and Christopher Stockton. 2003. "The Impact of the Flexner Report on the Fate of Medical Schools in North America after 1909." *Journal of American Physicians and Surgeons* 8 (2): 4.

9. Bierring, W. 1934. "The Family Doctor and the Changing Order." *Journal of the American Medical Association* 102:1995–98.

10. Starr, Paul. 1982. *The Social Transformation of American Medicine*, 421. New York: Basic Books.

11. Charter, GMENAC, Secretary David Mathews, April 20, 1976. Federal Register Vol. 41 No. 98, May 19, 1976. Quoted in McNutt, D. R. 1981. "GMENAC: Its Manpower Forecasting Framework." *American Journal of Public Health* 71 (10): 1116–24.

12. McNutt, D. R. 1981. "GMENAC: Its Manpower Forecasting Framework." *American Journal of Public Health* 71 (10): 1116–24.

13. Cooper, R. A., T. E. Getzen, H. J. McKee, and P. Laud. 2002. "Economic and Demographic Trends Signal an Impending Physician Shortage." *Health Affairs (Millwood)* 21 (1): 140–54.

14. Cooper, R. A. 2002. "There's a Shortage of Specialists: Is Anyone Listening?" *Academic Medicine* 77 (8): 761–66.

15. "New Research Shows Increasing Physician Shortages in Both Primary and Specialty Care." *AAMC News*, April 11, 2018. https://news.aamc.org/press-releases /article/workforce_report_shortage_04112018/.

16. Saltarelli, A. J., C. J. Roseth, and W. A. Saltarelli. 2014. "Human Cadavers vs. Multimedia Simulation: A Study of Student Learning in Anatomy." *Anatomical Sciences Education* 7 (5): 331–39. doi:10.1002/ase.1429.

17. Biasutto, S. N., L. I. Caussa, and L. E. Criado del Río. 2006. "Teaching Anatomy: Cadavers vs. Computers?" *Annals of Anatomy* 188 (2): 187–90.

18. Winkelmann, A. 2007. "Anatomical Dissection as a Teaching Method in Medical School: A Review of the Evidence." *Medical Education* 41 (1): 15–22.

19. Stillman, P. L., M. B. Regan, M. Philbin, and H. L. Haley. 1990. "Results of a Survey on the Use of Standardized Patients to Teach and Evaluate Clinical Skills." *Academic Medicine* 65 (5): 288–92.

20. Sklar, D. P. 2018. "Can Words on the Screen Replace the Face in the Classroom? Using the Internet to Revolutionize Medical Education." *Academic Medicine* 93 (8): 1095–97.

21. Barrows, H. S. 1968. "Simulated Patients in Medical Teaching." *Canadian Medical Association Journal* 98 (14): 674–78.

22. Barrows, H. S. 1983. "Problem-Based, Self-Directed Learning." *Journal of the American Medical Association* 250 (22): 3077–80.

23. Shea, C. A., and P. F. Plunkett. 2001. "Forum for Organizational Change in Health Professions Education: Summary of the Academic Organizational Approaches to Transforming Health Science Education Conference." *Journal of Interprofessional Care* 15 (3): 297–99.

24. Ford, C. D., P. G. Patel, V. S. Sierpina, M. W. Wolffarth, and J. L. Rowen. 2018. "Longitudinal Continuity Learning Experiences and Primary Care Career Interest: Outcomes from an Innovative Medical School Curriculum." *Journal of General Internal Medicine* 33 (10): 1817–21. doi:10.1007/s11606-018-4600-x.

25. Beran, R. L. 1979. "The Rise and Fall of Three-Year Medical School Programs." *Journal of Medical Education* 54 (3): 248–49.

26. Leong, S. L., et al. 2017. "Roadmap for Creating an Accelerated Three-Year Medical Education Program." *Medical Education Online* 22 (1): 1396172. doi:10.10 80/10872981.2017.1396172.

27. Silver, H. K., and A. D. Glicken. 1990. "Medical Student Abuse: Incidence, Severity, and Significance." *Journal of the American Medical Association* 263 (4): 527–32.

28. Cook, A. F., V. M. Arora, K. A. Rasinski, F. A. Curlin, and J. D. Yoon. 2014. "The Prevalence of Medical Student Mistreatment and Its Association with Burnout." *Academic Medicine* 89 (5): 749–54. doi:10.1097/ACM.0000000000000204.

29. Fried, J. M., M. Vermillion, N. H. Parker, and S. Uijtdehaage. "Eradicating Medical Student Mistreatment: A Longitudinal Study of One Institution's Efforts." *Academic Medicine* 87 (9): 1191–98.

30. Fnais, N., C. Soobiah, M. H. Chen, E. Lillie, L. Perrier, M. Tashkhandi, S. E. Straus, M. Mamdani, M. Al-Omran, and A. C. Tricco. 2014. "Harassment and Discrimination in Medical Training: A Systematic Review and Meta-analysis." *Academic Medicine* 89 (5): 817–27. doi:10.1097/ACM.0000000000000200.

31. Binder, R., P. Garcia, B. Johnson, and E. Fuentes-Afflick. 2018. "Sexual Harassment in Medical Schools: The Challenge of Covert Retaliation as a Barrier to Reporting." *Academic Medicine* 93 (12): 1770–73. doi:10.1097/ACM.0000000000002302.

32. Carr, P., C. M. Gunn, S. A. Kaplan, A. Raj, and K. M. Freund. "Inadequate Progress for Women in Academic Medicine: Findings from the National Faculty Study." *Journal of Women's Health* 24 (3): 190–99. doi:10.1089/jwh.2014.4848.

33. Nunez-Smith, M., M. M. Ciarleglio, T. Sandoval-Schaefer, J. Elumn, L. Castillo-Page, P. Peduzzi, and E. H. Bradley. 2012. "Institutional Variation in the Promotion of Racial/Ethnic Minority Faculty at US Medical Schools." *American Journal of Public Health* 102 (5): 852–58. doi:10.2105/AJPH.2011.300552.

34. Weiner, B. J., T. C. Ricketts III, E. P. Fraher, D. Hanny, and L. D. Coccodrilli. 2005. "Area Health Education Centers: Strengths, Challenges, and Implications for Academic Health Science Center Leaders." *Health Care Management Review* 30 (3): 194–202.

35. Acosta, D., and P. Olsen. 2006. "Meeting the Needs of Regional Minority Groups: The University of Washington's Programs to Increase the American Indian and Alaskan Native Physician Workforce." *Academic Medicine* 81 (10): 863–70.

36. Toney, M. 2012. "The Long, Winding Road: One University's Quest for Minority Health Care Professionals and Services." *Academic Medicine* 87 (11): 1556–61. doi:10.1097/ACM.0b013e31826c97bd.

37. Winkleby, M. A. 2007. "The Stanford Medical Youth Science Program: 18 Years of a Biomedical Program for Low-Income High School Students." *Academic Medicine* 82 (2): 139–45.

38. Thompson, H. C., III, and M. A. Weiser. 1999. "Support Programs for Minority Students at Ohio University College of Osteopathic Medicine." *Academic Medicine* 74 (4): 390–92.

39. Garces, L. M., and D. Mickey-Pabello. "Racial Diversity in the Medical Profession: The Impact of Affirmative Action Bans on Underrepresented Student of Color Matriculation in Medical Schools." *Journal of Higher Education* 86 (2): 264–94. doi:10.1353/jhe.2015.0009.

40. Thomas, B. R., and N. Dockter. 2019. "Affirmative Action and Holistic Review in Medical School Admissions: Where We Have Been and Where We Are Going." *Academic Medicine* 94 (4): 473–76. doi:10.1097/ACM.0000000000002482.

41. Thornton, R. L., C. M. Glover, C. W. Cené, D. C. Glik, J. A. Henderson, and D. R. Williams. 2016. "Evaluating Strategies for Reducing Health Disparities by Addressing the Social Determinants of Health." *Health Affairs (Millwood)* 35 (8): 1416–23. doi:10.1377/hlthaff.2015.1357.

42. Maeshiro, R., D. Koo, and C. W. Keck. 2011. "Integration of Public Health into Medical Education." *American Journal of Preventive Medicine* 41 (4 Suppl. 3): S145–48.

43. Strasser, R., P. Worley, F. Cristobal, D. Marsh, S. Berry, S. Strasser, and R. Ellaway. 2015. "Putting Communities in the Driver's Seat: The Realities of Community-Engaged Medical Education." *Academic Medicine* 90 (11): 1466–70.

44. Mariam, D. H., et al. "Community-Based Education Programs in Africa: Faculty Experience within the Medical Education Partnership Initiative (MEPI) Network." *Academic Medicine* 89 (8 Suppl.): S50–54.

45. White, K. L., T. F. Williams, and B. G. Greenberg. 1961. "The Ecology of Medical Care." *New England Journal of Medicine* 265:885–92.

46. White, K. 1973. "Life and Death and Medicine." *Scientific American* 229 (3): 23–33.

47. Green, L. A., G. E. Fryer Jr., B. P. Yawn, D. Lanier, and S. M. Dovey. 2001. "The Ecology of Medical Care Revisited." *New England Journal of Medicine* 344 (26): 2021–25.

48. Shannon, S. C., S. M. Ferretti, D. Wood, and T. Levitan. 2010. "The Challenges of Primary Care and Innovative Responses in Osteopathic Education." *Health Affairs (Millwood)* 29 (5): 1015–22. doi:10.1377/hlthaff.2010.0168.

49. Rabinowitz, H. K., J. J. Diamond, F. W. Markham, and A. J. Santana. 2013. "Retention of Rural Family Physicians after 20–25 Years: Outcomes of a Comprehensive Medical School Rural Program." *Journal of the American Board of Family Medicine* 26 (1): 24–27. doi:10.3122/jabfm.2013.01.120122.

50. MacDowell, M., M. Glasser, and M. Hunsaker. 2013. "A Decade of Rural Physician Workforce Outcomes for the Rockford Rural Medical Education (RMED) Program, University of Illinois." *Academic Medicine* 88 (12): 1941–47. doi:10.1097/ACM.0000000000000031.

51. Greysen, S. R., C. Chen, and F. Mullan. 2011. "A History of Medical Student Debt: Observations and Implications for the Future of Medical Education." *Academic Medicine* 86 (7): 840–45. doi:10.1097/ACM.0b013e31821daf03.

52. Murr, A. H., C. Miller, and M. Papadakis. 2002. "Mentorship through Advisory Colleges." *Academic Medicine* 77 (11): 1172–73.

53. Taylor, J. S., S. Faghri, N. Aggarwal, K. Zeller, R. Dollase, and S. P. Reis. "Developing a Peer-Mentor Program for Medical Students." *Teaching and Learning in Medicine* 25 (1): 97–102. doi:10.1080/10401334.2012.741544.

54. Kosoko-Lasaki O., R. E. Sonnino, and M. L. Voytko. 2006. "Mentoring for Women and Underrepresented Minority Faculty and Students: Experience at Two Institutions of Higher Education." *Journal of the National Medical Association* 98 (9): 1449–59.

55. Osterberg, L. G., E. Goldstein, D. S. Hatem, K. Moynahan, and R. Shochet. 2016. "Back to the Future: What Learning Communities Offer to Medical Education." *Journal of Medical Education and Curricular Development* 3:JMECD.S39420. doi:10.4137/JMECD.S39420.

56. Johnson, J. A., and K. Sekar. 2019. *National Institutes of Health (NIH) Funding: FY1994–FY2019.* Congressional Research Service. https://fas.org/sgp/crs/misc/R43341.pdf.

57. Morris, Z. S., S. Wooding, and J. Grant. 2011. "The Answer Is 17 Years, What Is the Question: Understanding Time Lags in Translational Research." *Journal of the Royal Society of Medicine* 104 (12): 510–20. doi:10.1258/jrsm.2011.110180.

58. Farley, T. A., M. A. Dalal, F. Mostashari, and T. R. Frieden. 2010. "Deaths Preventable in the U.S. by Improvements in the Use of Clinical Preventive Services." *American Journal of Preventive Medicine* 38 (6): 600–609.

The eight appendixes constitute a tool kit derived from the many projects guided by the Morehouse Model. These tools and resources are user-friendly products for those seeking to implement community engagement programs in their respective communities. A brief overview description is presented for each item, detailing the purpose, application, and audience as appropriate. These tools are only a subset of the vast array of tools that have been used by our program implementers.

A. Coalition Building Manual

The Coalition Building Manual is a document complied by Pat Thompson Reid, MPH, a former staff associate within the Health Promotion Research Center. The manual was developed from the original work on community empowerment as conceptualized by the HPRC founders in 1988–89. As noted in chapter 1, the initial test site community (Joyland/High Point) utilized the process and procedures for organizing this coalition. The manual has served as a blueprint for organizing and training numerous urban and rural communities for health promotion projects at the community level. The manual is intended to be used as a guide for unorganized groups interested in becoming a coalition. Specifically, the manual addresses (1) Coalition Building Processes, Strategies, and Issues; (2) Planning Community Interventions; (3) Implementing Community-Based Programs; and (4) Maintaining and Sustaining Coalitions. The manual is most effectively used by community organizers or community health workers in conjunction with a critical mass of community residents working side by side.

B. Coalition Training Needs Assessment

The coalition training needs assessment was developed by Braithwaite, Murphy, Blumenthal, and Lynthcott in 1989 as a tool to ascertain perceived areas for training and technical assistance among coalition members. The survey presents 35 training areas and asks the members to rate from low to high their perceived training needs. While the list of training areas is not an exhaustive list, it represents areas for training essential to the healthy growth and development of new coalitions. The training sessions were implemented on a monthly basis in conjunction with the monthly coalition board meeting. Typically, the coalition would use the first hour for coalition business, followed by the training sessions during the second hour of a two-hour coalition meeting. Both university and local resource persons are recruited to serve as topical area training presenters or facilitators. These training sessions are viewed as empathy-building activities critical to coalition sustainability.

C. Post-Workshop Evaluation Form

Everybody has experienced or been asked to complete a workshop evaluation form following a formal seminar, training, or workshop session. Use of such instruments is typical as a feedback mechanism for the program managers and training facilitator. These forms can take on many formats, including Likert scales, open-ended questions, and item rating formats. These instruments typically ask questions about the session format, the content, the physical environment, the presenters, and whether the stated session objectives are met. The respondent is often queried on what they liked most and least about the session. The instruments are usually developed by the local staff, who are able to tailor the question to a specific topical area. The respondent results are aggregated and used for planning future sessions, which are modified based on the nature of the feedback.

D. Community Health Needs Assessment Survey

The Morehouse School of Medicine Prevention Research Center Community Health Needs Assessment is conducted at least once every four years with community stakeholders. A community-based participatory approach is designed to use this tool to (1) identify the health needs, priorities, and perceptions to inform research and intervention implementation and (2) make recommendations for planning and implementing research projects, disease prevention activities, health promotion outreach, and evaluation initiatives in support of a community-based participatory research agenda. Core research and other strategically aligned projects are developed and implemented in response to priorities identified through these assessments. The CBPR-driven CHNA process and tool have implications for data-driven public health practice that is community owned and sustained. See chapter 6 for details on the community training and leadership strategies central to the planning, implementation, and evaluation central to conducting or adapting this approach.

E. Windshield Survey Process

The windshield survey process is not new and has been used by many working in the community organizing space. The process involves driving through a community or walking through a community to observe community dynamics.

F. Coalition Member Satisfaction Scale

The MSM PRC annually conducts the Community Coalition Board Satisfaction Survey among its members, a community-majority governing board to steer, rather than advise, CBPR and other community-engaged initiatives. The CCB has served as the *governing body* for the MSM PRC since the center's founding in 1999. The CCB bylaws stipulate that neighborhood representatives will always be in the majority on the board and that the board chair, vice chair, and secretary (not academic faculty/staff) will always be neighborhood representatives. Hence, in any vote that pits the neighborhoods against the academics and public health professionals, the neighborhoods would have the most votes (however, this has never occurred).

More than an assessment that sits on a shelf or in a virtual file, this tool is used to provide an evidence base for strategic action planning. It informs academic accountability toward annual reflection on the *pulse*, *temperature*, and *relationship* between the academic institution (faculty and staff at MSM) and the community members (residents, organizations, and agencies) who serve on the board. The assessment is strategically administered in June of each year to allow time for analysis, presentation, and time for discussion and reflection at an annual retreat in August. Surveys are completed face-to-face or electronically, based on board member preference. They are anonymous. The sample questions included in appendix F are each followed by a box for open-ended comments and for sharing any additional feedback. A community-academic co-led committee called Data Monitoring and Evaluation, established and active since 2011, analyzes and prepares results for retreat discussion. At the retreat, scores for each question in each priority area are compared to those of the prior year to identify areas of growth, change, or challenge. Reasons for changes in any direction (better or worse) are brainstormed for the purpose of developing plans for sustained improvements.

G. Medical Student–Developed Surveys

Medical students at MSM are required to take a community health education course. One of the course requirements is for the students to develop a small-scale group project that involves conducting a community survey on a small sample of community residents. A few of these medical student–developed surveys are included in appendix G.

H. Faculty Community Engagement Publication List

This appendix is composed of a list of publications by MSM faculty whose work focuses on CE. Specifically, the criterion for listing a publication was that it involved the use of a community coalition or involved a linkage or partnership effort with community constituents. Some of the publications report on CBPR projects or interpretation that had a collaborative as a central component.

Coalition Building Manual

Compiled by Pat Thompson-Reid, MPH

A Guide to Building Community Coalitions for Health Promotion

Table of Contents

The HPRC Approach

The Health Promotion Resource Center (HPRC) at the Morehouse School of Medicine was established in 1988 with a grant from the Kaiser Family Foundation with the primary goal of developing a health promotion and disease prevention model for minority communities.

The philosophy of the HPRC is that health promotion efforts are likely to be more successful in populations where the community at risk is empowered to identify its own health concerns, develop its own prevention and/or intervention strategies, and form a decision-making coalition board to make policy decisions and identify resources for program implementation.

The HPRC implements a community organization and development approach survey through the use of community organizers and other support staff. The primary role of community organizers is to build coalitions in urban and rural communities. This enables them to become more self-sufficient and empowers them to address health and other problems as they see fit. The process for achieving this involves

- the development of a demographic, socioeconomic, and epidemiologic profile;
- community entry;
- the organization of a consumer-dominated board/coalition;
- incorporation and nonprofit status;
- the implementation of a community health needs assessment;
- resource mobilization;
- planning and programming; and
- the implementation of a health intervention program.

Inherent in this process is the education of the coalition board and the transfer of management and operational skills for successful community-based programs. This is an ongoing process with participatory dialogue from the bottom up and the top down. It is through this type of exchange that the HPRC has been able to develop training programs and provide technical assistance that is relevant and successful in preparing the coalition boards for their tasks.

With funding from the Kaiser Family Foundation, the HPRC implemented this effort in two urban and two rural communities, as well as 28 additional communities throughout Georgia. A grant from the Center for Substance Abuse Prevention provided the funds to organize coalitions in 10 other counties to address substance abuse. The guide presented here is based on the experiences of the staff in facilitating this model for health promotion.

Purpose of the Guide

This manual is divided into five (5) parts. The historical background provides a brief perspective of the health status of our communities and the thinking that led to the recognition of coalition building as a strategy for health promotion. There is also a definition of important terms and a discussion of recent trends in health promotion.

The section titled "Coalition-Building Processes and Strategies" discusses the various components of the HPRC approach. Each step in the process is examined with emphasis on the most appropriate approach for achieving specific outcomes. This section is written from the perspective of an outsider who has entered a community to facilitate coalition building.

"Planning for Community Intervention Programs" discusses the planning process. It includes important activities such as the community needs assessment survey, the setting of priorities, resource mobilization, and the development of an intervention strategy.

"Implementing a Community-Based Program" addresses project management and the importance of management functions and structures. The development of guidelines and the importance of monitoring and evaluation are emphasized.

"Coalition Maintenance" deals with the events and processes that must be in place in order to provide continuity for community involvement and maintenance of the coalition.

This model for coalition building is one of many being developed by the HPRC in several communities. The ideas presented here are a result of the collective experience of the staff of the HPRC. The experience one could gain from this process would depend on his or her community, its history and current challenges, and one's degree of flexibility and responsiveness to the members the community.

Coalition-Building Processes and Strategies

I. Know Your Community

DEMOGRAPHIC, SOCIOECONOMIC, AND VITAL STATISTICS DATA
Before entering the community, the community organizer/health educator should become oriented to some basic facts about his/her target area. Demographic, socioeconomic, and vital statistics data will provide a general description of the target population and its activities, as well as provide indicators of morbidity and mortality.

FAMILIARIZATION WITH GEOGRAPHIC LOCATION
A telephone call to the state or local planning unit, the Chamber of Commerce, or the public transportation office will provide important information on the size and geographic features of the area, as well as the location and availability of public transportation facilities. Zoning maps can be secured from the city planning departments. The demarcation of census tracts for the catchment area to be targeted provides vital information on political districts. This would assist in defining the administrative and political units such as health districts and voting constituencies set up by the local government. The identification of historical landmarks, housing profiles, and the location of all service organizations should also be ascertained.

CULTURAL ECOLOGICAL STUDY OF COMMUNITY
Learning the community firsthand is essential in the process of coalition building. One must become familiar with the daily activities and rhymes of the

target area and the public transportation system and its users. Also important are the location and programs offered at the schools, churches, and health care and recreation centers.

It is also advantageous to visit the community at different times of the day in order to understand its cycles. What times do children return from school? Parents from work? What do most members of the community do on Saturdays? Where do the men in the community gather? What after-school activities do children participate in? Participation in various activities on holidays and weekends will also provide additional insight into the community and its social structure. Written notes should be made of when and where different groups of people gather, what they do together, and who the leaders are among them. In doing this, one must be cognizant of his/her safety and the community's attitude toward his/her presence. If it is a very closed community—one that does not accept outsiders very easily—then it may be wise to consult community leaders on the best approach to achieve this end.

II. Community Entry Process

COMMUNITY LEADERS

It is important to enter the community as tactfully as possible. Prior to entering the community, the community organizer* must identify and meet with the community leaders or the formal and informal gatekeepers of the neighborhood. These are the politicians, the ministers, the heads of community agencies, or the heads of local community groups, or outspoken community members who are respected by their peers. They are the decision-makers and consensus builders within their milieu. They are members of the community who know each other well and can influence one way or the other the success of the community entry process.

It is important for the community organizer to discuss the concerns of said gatekeepers and determine their opinions on how these concerns could best be addressed. These individuals will also be able to introduce you to other members of the community's leadership and facilitate the organization of community meetings and activities. Activities implemented without community consensus are an encroachment; therefore, the community organizer must be attuned to the cultural setting he or she has entered. He or she must accept the ideas and solutions offered by community members as meaningful based on the collective experience of the community.

COMMUNICATION WITH COMMUNITY MEMBERS

Communication with community members is very important during the community entry process and throughout the coalition-building initiative. The community's

---

*Could be health educator, social worker, and so forth. CO used conveniently throughout text.

culture will dictate its forms of expression. In some parts of the country it may be very important that a community organizer be cognizant of language differences such as dialects that may or may not affect communication. One should also keep in mind that the similarities between the community organizer and community members are normally greater than the differences. This means that important differences may go unnoticed. It is therefore important to study and be aware of these differences in order to avoid social embarrassment.

One of the most important factors in gaining the confidence of community members is sincerity. However, there will be times when we the "experts" feel frustrated because no matter how sincere we are, our knowledge is not understood or accepted. It may be that the communication has been on a one-way street. It is important to listen in the first instance and encourage dialogue so that communication can be initiated freely by either party. We are always eager to impart our knowledge to the community, but it may be not accepted. In many cases it will be resisted if not well thought out or timely. The community organizer is not effective until he/she can prove his/her worth on a purely human basis. This involves free and open communication with community members and participation in activities and events acceptable to them.

HOME VISITS

Home visits are encouraged only when invited. The community organizer should be cautious about making home visits until community-wide acceptance and rapport are established.

COMMUNITY DEVELOPMENT ACTIVITIES

As stated above, the community organizer/professional must tactfully choose to participate in or support community activities that are not only visible but also appropriate (i.e., Kwanzaa and various other Christmas celebrations, health fairs, community fairs, church-sponsored activities, little league games, and basketball games). No matter what the activity, the community organizer should only attend an activity if invited—activities that will allow him or her to interact with community members and allow them to get to know him/her and accept his/her presence. If possible, volunteering expertise in specific areas or accessing information on behalf of community members will enable the community organizer to prove his worth and also build credibility.

For most who have done community development work, the common complaint received from the community residents is that there is too much talk, too many surveys, too many promises, and too little action. There is always suspicion when the coalition is initiated by an outsider. This historical perspective gives community members a healthy cynicism that will influence the ability to evaluate the credibility of what is being communicated to them.

The professional must listen and observe his community and strive to integrate himself with the internal communications system already in place. This is why it is so very important to get to know the community and its people. For instance, it is important to pay attention to persons whose advice is sought more often than others and whose pronouncements are heeded. These community members influence the thoughts and decisions of many community members.

If and when the professional and his ideas are accepted, he/she can then assist and facilitate community development efforts with the least amount of presence through the assistance of community leaders. The community organizer must assist the community in

- identifying its own problems and needs;
- developing a plan for securing resources to meet needs;
- planning activities and projects to meet them;
- sharing and summarizing the experience of implementation;
- evaluating the causes of failure or success;
- incorporating the results of evaluation into the planning of new activities; and
- growing in skills and know-how in order to sustain independent community development efforts.

Instead of imposing predetermined plans on the community, the community organizer should assure community members that they are a part of the planning and decision-making process. They should be involved at all levels no matter how small or large the project or activity—from the point of conception to planning, implementation, and evaluation. By becoming involved, by defining the problem, and by taking ownership of the problem community members will become integrated in the process for eventually developing strategies for intervention.

The ultimate goal is for community members to become more conscious of their potential as human beings so that they can define their own needs, set their own priorities, choose their own solutions, and evaluate and monitor their successes and failures. This will not happen overnight but is part of an ongoing process more formally known as "empowerment."

III. Formation of the Coalition

The formation of a successful coalition by community members should be implemented when certain specific factors are in place. These include agreement on the existence of a general problem or set of problems, an expressed need from the community to attempt to impact the problems, and a consensus on the need for a mechanism to ensure a group approach to problem-solving. These factors increase the chances of the coalition being successful. When they are realized, it is then feasible for community members to consider the formation of a coalition board.

The recommended coalition composition is a board that is at least 75 percent consumer dominated, with the other 25 percent being representative of diverse health and human services organizations that serve the community (e.g. local chambers of commerce, United Way, third-party reimbursement organizations, pharmacists, lawyers, nurses, physicians, and others from the helping professions). Who should be invited to be on the board? Should there be politicians on the board? How does the core group appoint members? Is there a criterion for board membership? What happens if someone important is left off? Are there competing factors in the community? Who is a consumer versus a provider? How many members should there be on the board? These are all important questions to be discussed by the founding members.

First of all, a list of potential board members should be made and discussed. The community organizer can lead these discussions and serve as a resource person, but the ultimate decisions about membership should be made by community members. It is important, however, to select members who will bring certain skills and expertise to the board, are committed to the goals and objectives of the group, and are willing to commit at least two years of service to the board. It is also important to keep in mind that individuals who have positive relationships with service and resource organizations, as well as the power brokers in the community, state, or principal locality, must also be considered seriously for board membership. These individuals will play a vital role in building partnerships and securing the necessary resources and support for the coalition and its community.

Once a list of potential members is drawn up, then official contact should be made by the founding members by either letter, phone, or a personal visit, whichever is most appropriate. A personal visit is always more effective in recruiting members. Once a potential member has accepted the invitation, then a letter of confirmation should be sent.

The board should be no larger than 21 persons, and, initially, 16 persons is ideal. It has been demonstrated that in the first year several members will drop out for a variety of reasons. By the end of that year, there may only be a core group of 10 persons who attend regularly; the others may remain members but are not usually as active as may be desirable.

There are others who are committed to the goals and objectives of the board and who will respond to specific needs of the board, but they are unable to attend regular meetings. These members should be cultivated as they may be of considerable value to the board. It is important, however, that they are kept abreast of the activities of the board at all times even though they are not present at all meetings. This can be achieved by sending minutes to absentee members on a regular basis.

The name and logo for the organization should be developed and a formal statement should be drafted stating the goals and objectives of the coalition. Election of officers could then take place, or, more appropriately, the election of officers could take place after the bylaws have been developed. The election of officers may be expedient before the development of bylaws in order to provide some structure to the newly founded organization and provide a means of establishing leadership for coalition activities.

THE BYLAWS

The internal regulations of the board are contained in its bylaws. In order to legitimize the internal structure of the organization, bylaws for the coalition should be developed and approved by coalition members, outlining the following:

1. Purpose
2. Composition
3. Duties of members
4. Voting rights and quorum
5. Standing committees
6. Frequency of meetings
7. Procedure for amending

This is a very important turning point for the community participation process. The formality legitimizes the process as the group becomes actively involved, mentally and physically, in a range of decision-making processes.

IV. Incorporation and Tax Exemption

The coalition should become incorporated. This makes the coalition a legal entity in the state in which it is formed. It also provides legal protection for individual members from lawsuits. In order to become incorporated, the newly formed coalition must decide on a name that is uniquely theirs and file a letter of incorporation in the office of the Secretary of State. This includes the goal and objectives of the corporation, its projected duration, and its bylaws. The number of directors and officers must also be listed.

These will vary from one state to another; therefore, it is important to check with the office of the Secretary of State in each state to determine the requirements for the incorporation of a nonprofit community agency. The coalition should also decide if it wants to apply for nontax status.[†]

V. The Structure of the Board

As previously stated, the election of officers provides leadership and structure to the newly formed organization. The board is made up of members who

---

[†]This provides exemption from certain state taxes, advance assurance to donors of deductibility of a contribution, exemption from certain federal excise taxes, and nonprofit mailing privileges. This process should begin shortly after the incorporation process and no more than 15 months after.

represent the community it serves. It is responsible for the development of policies and projects and the selection of personnel to carry out the function as well as objectives of the coalition. In order to facilitate this process, officers must be elected, and chairpersons of standing committees should also be elected or appointed by the executive committee of the board.

Chairperson or President. The chairperson's basic responsibility is to preside over the board and maintain order, to announce all business, to be informed on all communications, and to be absolutely fair and impartial.

Vice President. In the absence of the president the vice president performs his/her duties.

Secretary. Keeps a record of attendance and the proceedings of all meetings. Above all else, this record should always reflect resolutions or motions adopted. These would form the minutes and are presented at regular meetings for adoption.

Treasurer. The treasurer is responsible for all funds received and all sums paid out. The treasurer should also report the balance at hand and expenditures at each meeting. An annual report should also be prepared at the end of the year.

VI. Formation of Standing Committees

The Executive Committee. The executive committee includes the officers of the coalition board and, if stated in the bylaws, the chairpersons of each standing committee. The executive committee strengthens the position of the president, conducts routine business between meetings, and acts in emergencies. In some cases, the president will appoint committee chairpersons upon recommendations from the executive committee.

Standing Committees. Standing committees are usually committees named in the bylaws and function throughout the year. These committees are given specific responsibilities in order to expedite the goals and objectives of the coalition and allow for participation by coalition members. These committees are also required to submit reports with recommendations to the full board for discussion and adoption. This is not a recipe for every board, as the ultimate decision for the formation of committees would be dependent on the need for which it functions.

Suggested standing committees are:

1. Finance
2. Program and planning
3. Personnel
4. Resource development
5. Public relations

Once the standing committees are decided on, the chairpersons for each committee can either be nominated and elected by the full board or be appointed by the chairperson. Volunteers should be drafted from board members based on their area of expertise.

Ad Hoc Committees. These committees are set up to perform a special task, secure more information, investigate a situation, and report back or present a recommendation to the full board. These are temporary committees that cease to function once the task is completed. However, because they can be varied and focus on different issues/projects, they provide opportunities for coalition members to become involved in areas of their particular interest.

VII. Coalition Board Training

It is important that members of the coalition board receive training so that they can be prepared for their new role. Without adequate training, members may not know how to perform in their role of policy and decision-makers. They may also fail to develop the confidence that is needed to achieve the objectives of the coalition. Initially this training might include the following:

1. Interpersonal relationships
2. The role and responsibilities of the board
3. Team building
4. Health promotion and intervention
5. Fiscal responsibility
6. Problem-solving

As the board progresses, other topics for board training could be:

1. Conflict resolution
2. Project management
3. Grassroots fundraising
4. Tax responsibilities of the board
5. Proposal writing
6. Board/staff relationships
7. Seminars on various issues affecting minorities

The initial training should be intensive. If funds are available, what has proven most effective is the selection of a training facility outside of the community so that all of the attention can be focused on the goals and objectives of the training exercise. The training should also include informal interaction among board members. This gives members a chance to relax and to get to know one another. It also gives the community organizer as well as the board members an opportunity to observe and interact with each other in formal and informal settings.

An annual retreat could also serve as a means of reviewing the progress of the board, as well as a venue for training board members in areas of need as identified by them, or as recommended by the community organizer.

Planning for Community Intervention Programs

I. Implementing a Community Health Needs Assessment Survey

The needs assessment is designed to assist the coalition board in identifying the community's perceived health needs and concerns. It can also provide a demographic profile of the community and important information on the knowledge, attitudes, and health practices of its members. Technical assistance should be provided to coalition board members by the community organizer or other experts, if necessary, in the design of the survey instrument, the determination of the appropriate sample size and methods, the training of interviewers, the cost of the entire process, and the analysis and presentation of results.

Due to the importance of this activity, lack of financial resources should not serve as a deterrent. If community members are convinced of the importance of the survey, creative solutions have proven successful in overcoming a shortage of funds. For example, coalition members may volunteer as interviewers for the survey. If the community is aware of the purpose of the survey, community members may be willing to participate in the process without requesting payment for their services.

Minority communities have been surveyed so many times without any follow-up of the results or how the information would be used that many communities are now reluctant to participate in any such activity. Once the importance of this process is conveyed to community members, however, it should be viewed as an important step in the community development process. The participation of community members is critical since they know what their problems are and their opinions are important.

In order to address issues of cultural diversity, the community's input in design refinement of the survey is of utmost importance. The following is a breakdown of the suggested components of the survey:

A. Demographic and socioeconomic information (i.e., sex, race, age, marital, and employment status).
B. Basic information on interviewees' health concerns.
C. Questions about interviewees' health practices (e.g., exercise, diet, smoking, drinking, health checkup).
D. Questions related to infectious and chronic diseases.
E. Questions related to other health concerns: violence, teen pregnancy, drug abuse, AIDS.
F. Questions designed to investigate interviewees' internal and external locus of control.

In order to maximize accuracy and compliance with this activity, the interview should not exceed 45 minutes to an hour. It is important that all interviewers are trained and, more importantly, that they are also familiar with the community and its members.

The results of the survey should be analyzed and presented appropriately to the coalition and to interested members of the community at a community forum. This would (1) involve coalition members and members of the community in the final phase of this activity, (2) facilitate discussion and ownership of the problems as outlined in the results, and (3) begin the process of prioritizing and planning for specific interventions that would address the health problems as identified in the community health needs assessment.

The health assessment survey is designed to examine the perceived health needs among members of the community. It is an important step in the process of empowerment, and it provides a basis for the planning and prioritizing of future health intervention activities.

II. Development of Priorities for Health Intervention

With the completion of the community needs assessment and the knowledge of the community and its people, the coalition board and community organizer can now begin to identify priority problems and select appropriate interventions to address them. During this process, all coalition board members must be given the opportunity to participate openly.

The results of the health needs assessment survey provide quantitative baseline information and also information that reflects community values, health beliefs, and practices. The staff support person should also be able to superimpose regional or county health status data to further substantiate and exemplify the findings of the survey. This legitimizes concerns, not so much for the benefit of the community members but for those outside the community who may be influential in providing support (technical, administrative, or monetary) in the resolution of the stated concerns.

Respondents in the survey can be asked to prioritize their health concerns. This is one means of getting maximum community participation in the process of prioritizing. However, if this is not done, then the prioritizing of health concerns is an important exercise for the coalition board, which represents the community. If the prioritizing of health concerns was already determined in the needs assessment, the emphasis would then be focused on ranking solutions to problems or the design for intervention.

This process must be well thought out in order to allow maximum participation and fairness. If several concerns or strategies are being considered, then all should be listed with the expected benefits and costs of each. All board members must receive copies of the list for the study and discussion at regular board meetings. No additions should be made by support staff once these lists have been agreed upon. It may be easier for the community organizer to present a proposal for intervention to the coalition; however, offering a "menu" of proposed interventions and going through the process of prioritizing and looking at the feasibility of all options provides the board with options for their consideration and, thereby, allows the coalition to retain control of solving its own problems.

III. Resource Mobilization

Concurrent with the process of defining and prioritizing health problems, the coalition board should begin to take an inventory of what resources are available to it. This factor will influence what the coalition will eventually be able to do in order to solve its problems. Factors to consider include

- the availability of space;
- the availability of equipment (this includes office supplies, furniture, vehicles);
- funding source by program area;
- the availability of volunteer professional services (grantsmanship, legal advice, nursing services, clergy counseling, job placement services, cooks, dietitians, carpentry, medical services, media specialist);
- local community businesses; and
- agencies providing services in the community.

The full participation of the board in the preparation of this list should be solicited. This would serve to widen the pool of volunteers. At the same time this list should also be approved by the board in order to get a consensus on whom to seek for services or for funds.

The board should also take stock of its monetary resources and decide on fundraising activities that would provide monies for the community activities such as Kwanzaa, Easter egg hunts, Breakfast with Santa, Halloween Trick or Treat, and also petty cash for stamps and official board meetings. Fundraising is an important activity to maintain, even if a major funding source is acquired in the future by the coalition.

IV. Development of the Intervention Strategy

Once the coalition has decided on a disease priority determined and supported by mortality and morbidity data as well as the community survey, the coalition is now ready to consider possible interventions to make an impact on the health problems of the community.

For example, the following numbered items are possible control strategies and the lettered items are possible interventions:

1. Controlling hypertension
   a. Identify and treat uncontrolled hypertension
   b. Increase level of awareness on the effects of hypertension
2. Maintaining ideal weight
   a. Weight reduction program
   b. Recreational program
   c. Nutritional education

3. Smoking cessation and prevention
    a. Smoking cessation program
    b. Smoking prevention in schools.

ACCESS FEASIBILITY

In order to maximize the use of available resources, each strategy must be addressed in the most effective and economical way. Is it economically or technically feasible to prevent or control this disease at the community level with existing resources? How much will the intervention cost? What programs are already in place? Are they capable of meeting the perceived or actual needs of the community? Where are the gaps? Can the efforts of the coalition be coordinated with existing programs to reduce the risk for the disease, or to effectively control the disease? Is it feasible to obtain resources to develop new programs? The community organizer should discuss in a systematic manner the risk factors associated with the disease and then look at the feasibility of each possible strategy to reduce this risk.

ACCESS IMPORTANCE: THE EXAMPLE OF HYPERTENSION

What is the prevalence of hypertension in the community? How does it compare to city, state, and national data? Are there serious health consequences exhibited in the community as a result of this problem? Should the same considerations be taken for smoking and ideal weight maintenance as control measures? What is the reaction of the community to these health problems that are influenced by their lifestyle and behavior? Are these behaviors dictated by culture? By poverty? Is the community very concerned or just a little concerned about them? If this is ignored in the planning process, the program intervention may fail.

Based on the community's interest, what is the likelihood of getting the community's participation in the suggested interventions? Are community members more likely to participate in a demonstration nutrition education program for weight control or a smoking cessation program? These consider-ations will help to determine the overall priority for each strategy and allow the board to make more objective decisions regarding its final selection.

SELECT PRIORITY GROUP

Are there any particular groups in the community that are more at risk than others? Are there sufficient resources to allow for community-wide participation in the project? Will the intervention concentrate on infants, youth, adults, or the elderly, or any combination of these? All of these factors should be considered openly by the board with support from the community organizer/health educator who can provide data that will assist in the final selection on priorities and the most appropriate target groups.

Once the strategy has been decided on and the target group has been identified, then one should look at what barriers could prevent the target population from following or complying with the activities identified for each strategy. Analysis of a list of what each target individual and health provider is expected to do should lead to a third list of those specific activities that may not be carried out due to attitudes, beliefs, obstacles, or skills and knowledge deficiencies. For an intervention to have an impact, these barriers must be addressed in the design of the intervention. There are three basic reasons that prevent people from complying with health promotion activities:

1. Lack of knowledge about illness or existing resources
2. Lack of access (no insurance, distance to service, lack of funds, problems with communication, language deficiencies)
3. Lack of motivation resulting from attitudes toward illness, culture, locus of control

Barriers must be examined not only for the target population but also from the perspective of the providers of services. The development of objectives for the intervention program should incorporate all of the above, taking into consideration the availability of resources in the community and the most appropriate technology for achieving program objectives.

Implementing a Community-Based Program

Once the board has reached a consensus on its intervention strategy with clearly stated goals and objectives and has acquired the necessary resources for implementation, then an implementation plan should be developed. This plan should outline clearly the goals and objectives of the project, the activities to be carried out for each component, the persons responsible for each action step, and the dates for the projected completion of the activity.

Intervention objectives should state how much and when problems should be affected by the intervention. For example, if controlling hypertension was chosen as the area for intervention, then a possible intervention objective would be to increase, by the following year, the number of diagnosed hypertensives receiving follow-up care by 50 percent.

In developing this plan, the board should also look into existing programs to avoid duplication and to determine if capacity building may not be an appropriate strategy, compared to the development of parallel programs. What will happen when the coalition's resources are expended? Will the services still exist in the community? This could entail meetings with existing service agencies to discuss the community's concern about its services and to determine where community resources and input can best be utilized. This exercise is also an opportunity to develop linkages and relationships with key persons in these agencies for future collaboration on other issues or programs.

It is also important at this time that an evaluation plan be instituted to monitor the progress of the project and to incorporate in the everyday workings of the project proper documentation or data collection procedures. This will facilitate the evaluation of the project at designated periods as stated in the implementation plan.

In preparing an implementation plan, it is important to pace program activities appropriately. It is also suggested that a pre-implementation period be incorporated into the plan. During this time, the board would prepare for its operational activities. The key policy-making units of the board that govern its operations must be in place and function effectively during this period. If staff is to be hired, then the personnel committee must develop and present to the full board personnel policies before the hiring of new staff. This is an important policy function that outlines to each new employee the rules and regulations for working with the organization.

The finance committee will also have greater responsibility as grant funds require special procedures for accountability and for the monitoring of expenditures. Several accounts may have to be established at banks designated by the board, contracts prepared and reviewed, and payroll as well as procedures for the procurement and payment of services established. The program and planning committee plays a major role in the development of the implementation plan and would work closely with all other committees in scheduling the timely implementation of activities.

The public relations committee would prepare materials for distribution to community members. It is important to keep the community aware and informed of the activities of the coalition. This will validate its mission and encourage full participation by the community.

It is also conceivable that some of these various tasks will be subcontracted to an outside firm or individual; nevertheless, the board and its committees must be cognizant of the importance of their roles and function and be sufficiently trained in these so that they can monitor the implementation of any task or activities that fall within their realm of responsibility.

Coalition Maintenance

The successful development and implementation of activities in the community, no matter how large or small the scale, is a positive learning experience for the coalition board, the staff, and the community at large. It assists in the generation of community-wide support for the coalition and provides positive reinforcement for the board and its staff.

In keeping with the process of empowerment, there should also be a concurrent transfer of technology through the reinforcement of basic management processes and skills. If a program or activity was unsuccessful in achieving its outcome, an opportunity exists to sit again at the planning table, to examine closely the program or activity, and to learn from the experience. What did we do wrong? How can we do better the next time? An examination of what was done and how it was done would be most effective in this exercise.

The most important factor in this process is community participation. No matter what the successes or failures, it is crucial to maintain a high level of participation from community members so that the coalition can survive.

There are four basic considerations for sustaining the life of a coalition:

1. Attitudinal and behavioral changes
2. Effective leadership
3. Monitoring and evaluation
4. Integration

I. Attitudinal and Behavioral Changes

In the early stages of coalition building there is information gathering on the part of the community organizer and the community members. The implementation of the needs assessment survey with full participation of the community is a means of transferring technology. At the same time, it allows participants to become more critically aware of their health status and needs. The planning process that follows provides an opportunity to define problems more clearly and discuss options for solving them—taking into consideration existing services and other potential resources.

There will also be indicators of need, aside from those projected for the community projects. An assessment of discrepancies between what the community knows and what the community does is important in identifying health education needs and objectives. Some of these needs can usually be met by training, which would form the content of the community health education curriculum.

The training of coalition board members, however, is an organizing effort that contributes to the learning of new skills, the acquisition of knowledge, improved communication, and eventually to changes in attitudes and practice among coalition members. By virtue of the fact that they are perceived as having access to valuable resources, board members will become more visible in the community and will normally be viewed in high esteem. This perception places added responsibility on board members and may, in fact, lead to conflict in small communities where proximity creates problems arising from personal/community relationships and professional/board responsibilities.

As a result of this, the educational content of the total program should not be confined to vocational or technical objectives but should also be extended to the development of knowledge and skills for leadership that include group dynamics, problem-solving, and the art of negotiation/conflict resolution. The training of coalition members should be an ongoing process with redefinition of roles as operational and policy issues arise. Training is a key element for the operation of a functional board. An important task of the community organizer is an assessment of these needs and the timely implementation of a training program.

The attitudes and behavior of the institutions involved in the coalition building process are also critical in achieving success. Some institutions may not be fully committed politically or operationally to the concept of empowerment. Neither may the institutions be fully committed to full participation by the community. This results in conflicts. In many cases, it is only through such conflict that one can effect change. It is here also that experiential or didactic exercises eventually lead to changes in behavior.

These factors also imply that the community organizer must be knowledgeable of the culture about his or her institution and the community in which he works. He/she must be aware of prevailing health beliefs and practices, the roles and responsibilities of each sector of the community, the community's leadership, and the political, economic, and social costs of recommended changes.

II. Effective Leadership

Leadership is defined as the ability to guide a group toward the achievement of its goal. In the formation of a coalition, one of the important tasks is the election of officers. This provides structure and hopefully leadership for the total organization. Initially, some community groups may elect as their leader the most educated or articulate individual, usually to combat the insecurities felt when dealing with individuals from outside the community. History demonstrates that unless these individuals encourage true participation from board members, they are usually considered status seekers and may not really be trusted. In some cases, they do not truly identify with the group and may not adequately represent their needs. Once the coalition is established, these persons are usually removed from office.

In coalition building for health promotion, the most effective leadership styles are those that are democratic, involve the group in decision-making, recognize each member's skills and contributions, enact agreed-upon policies, and promote the interest of the group. The leader of the group should be involved in either task or group maintenance activities and maintain open communication with its constituents at all times. The establishment of effective communication can be achieved through genuine friendliness, mutual respect, knowledge, and trust of oneself and each other.

It is also important that the community organizer, or the person providing technical assistance, not become an officer on the coalition board. This results in too much dependence on this individual and will prevent the widening of the view of the coalition's role in community development. The coalition board may restrict itself only to questions dealing with health or whatever sector the community organizer represents. External assistance should be provided only if members need the knowledge, skill, or resource to accomplish what they have to do. Once this need is fulfilled, the community organizer should be able to gradually withdraw his or her presence from the community. It is important for the coalition to become independent as soon as possible, with the knowledge that its members can seek assistance whenever they deem it necessary.

III. Monitoring and Evaluation

The evaluation of the coalition board and its achievement and the evaluation of its intervention projects are important activities to be undertaken. During the process of coalition building, the board has to complete several steps in order to become a recognized entity. How long did this process take, and what were the restricting factors? Each community has its own unique set of problems and personalities—the documentation of the coalition-building process is an important activity. The community organizer should keep a log of this process and document meetings, dates, special concerns, and breakthrough events. For example, when was the first meeting conducted by a community person? When and how did each officer of the board take on his/her responsibilities? When did the board implement its first community activity? How many persons attended, and was the event successful?

In keeping with the principles of empowerment, issues relating to the board and its perception of itself and its relationship with the community-at-large should be analyzed. Has the board taken ownership of the problems in the community? Has it begun to examine or to mobilize resources to solve these problems? Is it able to effectively manage these resources? Criteria for measuring empowerment have yet to be developed. Until such time, however, we can begin to document the process and note the various patterns that emerge.

As stated before in the development of the intervention strategy, an evaluation plan must be an integral part of program development. Evaluation needs must be well thought out. Are there tests to be conducted? Data to be collected? What are the planning products? When were they completed? Also important are the resources to achieve the evaluation. Is there a special evaluator assigned to the project, or are evaluation activities an integral part of the everyday tasks of the project staff? How often will formal evaluations be done?

Time and resource considerations are important in planning for evaluation activities. It is also important that before any evaluation is done, baseline data are collected so that the results of the intervention can be compared with status before the intervention. Evaluation serves three basic purposes:

1. To monitor whether program objectives are being met
2. To document the appropriateness, effectiveness, and utilization of activities/services

3. To document the program for accountability to the community, for funding sources, and for replication by others

There are also three basic types of evaluation that will assist in assessing the achievement of intervention objectives.

Outcome evaluation is designed to evaluate the long-term health outcomes anticipated by conducting an intervention within a specific target population. It must be conducted long enough after the intervention has been initiated for behavioral changes and other factors to affect the outcome. Rates for death and illness are the traditional measures of health status for specific diseases. This is often very difficult to evaluate, as the outcome may not be apparent for many years after the project has ended.

Impact evaluation is designed to determine if an intervention's objective has been achieved or assesses to what extent an intervention strategy is effective in changing knowledge, attitudes, and behaviors.

Process evaluation is the documentation of the implementation of the intervention. It indicates what was done and how it was done. This should be an ongoing review of activities that can be achieved with daily logs or structured monthly reports. The results of an evaluation will help the board to assess the effectiveness of the intervention strategy and to determine if and when changes can be made to improve it.

IV. Integration

The continued success of the coalition is dependent on its ability to integrate itself into the socioeconomic and political environment within and outside of the community. The coalition and its leadership must build partnerships with other agencies with similar needs and interests or at least seek to create an atmosphere for interagency cooperation.

There will be many problems identified during the community organization process where community needs cross sectorial lines. For example, if substance abuse is considered a priority problem, then the schools may have to play a part (education), as must the hospital (health), drug or treatment center (rehabilitation), job training (business and labor), or the church (religious sector). All or some of these sectors may have to work together to make an impact on the problem. If efforts to bring about change are coordinated, then, in fact, there will be a more efficient use of resources and, beyond that, a more holistic approach to the problem.

Ideally, the community level is the most appropriate place for the integration of activities because it is only here where the smallest unit of any operational entity can interact with other entities to maximize efforts and bring about change. At the macro level, bureaucracies tend to be authoritarian, paternalistic, and territorial—all of which serve as barriers toward cooperation and collaboration. Knowledge and skills in the mobilization of resources both external and internal must be acquired. This knowledge, good leadership, the commitment of community members to take on solvable and appropriate problems, their mutual respect for each other, and shared responsibility are all important ingredients for successful coalitions and healthy communities.

The coalition can serve several functions in the community. It can serve as a conduit for information and resource sharing and also provide a pool of expertise in several areas. Coalition members should also sit on other boards that serve the community so that they can influence policy at all levels. Most importantly, coalition board members should—within their own authority—plan and coordinate services in the community, set policy, and act as an advocate for the people they serve.

Community Coalition Member Training

Needs Assessment Survey

Purpose

The purpose of this survey is to determine areas of needed training to enhance planning and coalition board member effectiveness.

Please check whether you have low or high need for training in the following areas:

(*see next page*)

	Low			High	
	1	2	3	4	5
1. Organizational Development					
2. Resource Development					
3. Leadership Skills					
4. Community Problem-Solving					
5. Project Management					
6. Fiscal Management					
7. Community Organization					
8. Coalition Member Recruitment Strategies					
9. Community Health Needs Assessment Survey					
10. Community Mobilization Strategies					
11. Nonprofit Incorporation					
12. IRS Tax-Exempt Status					
13. Effective Meeting Management					
14. Communication Skills					
15. Dealing with the Media					
16. Selecting/Developing Health Interventions					
17. Substance Abuse Prevention Programs					
18. Proposal Development					
19. Conflict Resolution					
20. Board-Staff Resolution					
21. Program Evaluation					
22. Supervising Staff Personnel					
23. Team Building					
24. Use of Consultants					
25. Obtaining Technical Assistance					
26. Interpersonal Communication					
27. Short-Range Planning					
28. Long-Range Planning					
29. Program Reporting					
30. Program Development					
31. Newsletter Development					
32. Other_____					
33. Other_____					
34. Other_____					

Workshop Evaluation Form

Workshop Title: _____

Today's Date: _____ Name of Presenter/s: _____

For the following areas, please indicate your rating with:

1 = Poor (P)　2 = Fair (F)　3 = Good (G)　4 = Excellent (E)

A. Content	(P)	(F)	(G)	(E)
Covered useful material	1	2	3	4
Practical to my needs and interests	1	2	3	4
Well organized	1	2	3	4
Well paced	1	2	3	4
Presented at the right level	1	2	3	4
Effective activities	1	2	3	4
Useful visual aids and handouts	1	2	3	4
B. Presentation	1	2	3	4
Instructor's knowledge	1	2	3	4
Instructor's presentation style	1	2	3	4
Instructor covered material clearly	1	2	3	4
Instructor responded well to questions	1	2	3	4
Instructor facilitated interactions among participants well	1	2	3	4
Overall, how would you rate this workshop?	1	2	3	4

A. What did you like most about this workshop?

B. What did you like least about this workshop?

C. How could this workshop be improved?

D. Any other comments or suggestions?

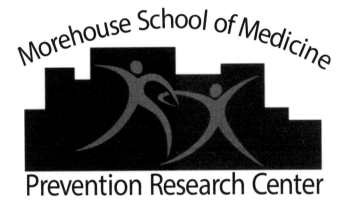

MSM PRC Community Health Needs & Assets Assessment Survey

The Morehouse School of Medicine Prevention Research Center is conducting a Community Health Needs and Assets Assessment. As a neighborhood resident of Neighborhood Planning Units (NPUs) T, V, X, Y, and Z, your opinion about the health concerns and resources in your community is important to us.

The information you give will help us develop health promotion programs and improve prevention education services that can benefit you and your family. Please take fifteen minutes of your time right now to complete this survey. Remember, there are no right or wrong answers and the information you provide will not be used to identify you. Please tell us what you think.

Before we begin—have you completed this survey already?

○ Yes
○ No
○ Not Sure

1 Which community do you live in? (Check One)

o Adair Park
o Amal Heights
o Ashview Heights
o Atlanta University Center
o Betmar La Villa
o Blair Villa/Poole Creek
o Browns Mill Park
o Capitol Gateway
o Capitol View
o Capitol View Manor
o Chosewood Park
o Glenrose Heights
o Hammond Park
o Harris Chiles
o High Point
o Joyland
o Just Us
o Lakewood
o Lakewood Heights
o Leila Valley

o Mechanicsville
o Norwood Manor
o Orchard Knob
o Peoplestown
o Perkerson
o Pittsburgh
o Polar Rock
o Rebel Valley Forest
o Rosedale Heights
o South Atlanta
o South River Gardens
o Summerhill
o Sylvan Hills
o The Villages at Carver
o The Villages at Castleberry Hill
o Thomasville Heights
o West End
o Westview
o Other (Please Specify) _____
o Don't Know

2 What Neighborhood Planning Unit (NPU) do you live in?
○ T
○ V
○ X
○ Y
○ Z
○ Other (Please Specify) _____
○ Don't Know

3 What is your zip code? _____

WE WOULD LIKE TO HEAR MORE ABOUT HEALTH CONCERNS IN YOUR COMMUNITY.

4 What are the <u>top **three** health issues my community needs to know</u> more about? **(Rank only three health issues by writing a "1" in the box next to the first priority, the second priority "2," and the third priority "3.") My community** needs to know more about:

	Ranking
Asthma	
Cancer	
Diabetes	
Environmental Health (e.g., air pollution, landfills, litter)	
Heart Disease	
High Blood Pressure	
HIV/AIDS	
Men's Health	
Mental Health	
Nutrition	
Obesity	
Physical Disability	
Second- or Thirdhand Smoke	
Sexually Transmitted Diseases or Infections (e.g., Chlamydia, Herpes, Gonorrhea, Syphilis)	
Stroke	
Substance Abuse	
Teen Pregnancy	
Violence Prevention	
Women's Health	
Other (Please List)	

5 For each of your top three choices, please tell us why the health issues you chose are important.

6 What do you think are the causes of the health issues/concerns you identified?

7 What do you think should be done to solve these health issues/concerns?

8 Please <u>rank the top three health issues you would like to learn more about for yourself.</u> **(Rank only three health issues by writing a "1" in the box next to the first priority, the second priority "2," and the third priority "3.")** For my **OWN** health, I want to learn more about:

	Ranking
Asthma	
Cancer	
Diabetes	
Environmental Health	
Heart Disease	
High Blood Pressure	
HIV/AIDS	
Men's Health	
Mental Health	
Nutrition	
Obesity	
Physical Disability	
Second- or Thirdhand Smoke	
Sexually Transmitted Diseases or Infections	
Stroke	
Substance Abuse	
Teen Pregnancy	
Violence Prevention	
Women's Health	
Other (Please List)	
_____	

9 For each of your top three choices, please tell us why the health issues you chose are important for you.

10 What are the top **three** policy, system, or environmental issues that need to be addressed in my community to improve health? **(Rank only three issues by writing a "1" in the box next to the first priority, the second priority "2," and the third priority "3.")** For my COMMUNITY, I want the following to be addressed:

	Ranking
Access to Health Insurance	
Access to Healthy Foods	
Access to the Internet/Technology	
Access to Physical Activity	
Access to Quality Healthcare Services	
Child Care	
Employment	
Health Education	

Housing	
Mental Health Treatment	
Poverty	
Public Education System	
Racism	
Sexism	
Substance Abuse	
Transportation	
Youth Employment	
Youth Engagement (e.g., Recreation Centers)	
Other (Please List) _____	

11 For each of your top three choices, please tell us why the policy, system, or environmental issues you chose are important.

NOW, WE WOULD LIKE TO KNOW WHAT HEALTH PROGRAMS AND SERVICES ARE AVAILABLE TO YOU

12 Are there any health programs in your community (e.g. walking clubs, weight loss programs)?
○ Yes (Please List) _____
○ No
○ Don't know

13 Have you attended any health programs in your community?
○ Yes (Please List) _____
○ No

14 The Morehouse School of Medicine Prevention Research Center has a number of community health programs for community members. We would like your input on how to let people know about these programs. Where do you think the top three places are to invite community members to hear about these programs? **(Please select three choices.)**
❏ Churches
❏ Community Events
❏ Daycare Centers
❏ Health Clinics
❏ Neighborhood Businesses
❏ Neighborhood Centers (Please specify name) _____

- ❏ Neighborhood Meetings
- ❏ Public Assistance Office
- ❏ Rental Offices
- ❏ School Meetings
- ❏ Other (Please List) _____

15 Do you have health insurance?
- ○ Yes
- ○ No (Skip to question 18)

16 If so, what? (Check all that apply.)
- ❏ Insurance through a current or former employer or union
- ❏ Insurance purchased directly from an insurance company
- ❏ Medicare, for people 65 and older, or people with certain disabilities
- ❏ Medicaid, Medical Assistance, or any kind of government-assistance plan for those with low incomes or a disability
- ❏ TRICARE or other military health care
- ❏ VA (including those who have ever used or enrolled for VA health care)
- ❏ Indian Health Service
- ❏ Grady Health card
- ❏ Any other type of health insurance or health coverage plan not listed (Please List) _____

17 If other, is your health insurance public or private?
- ○ Public
- ○ Private

18 Do you have supplemental insurance (i.e., additional insurance that pays directly to the insured such as AFLAC)?
- ○ Yes
- ○ No

19 Do you have a primary care doctor?
- ○ Yes
- ○ No

20 Do you participate in any of the following activities to prevent poor health?
- ❏ Eat healthy foods
- ❏ Exercise daily on a regular basis
- ❏ Receive annual flu shot

- ❏ See the dentist for routine dental exams
- ❏ See the doctor for annual physical exams
- ❏ Take a daily multivitamin or mineral supplement
- ❏ Take children to receive scheduled shots (immunization)
- ❏ Other (Please list)

21 Do you primarily seek health care in an emergency room?
- ○ Yes
- ○ No

22 Where do you usually get health care? (Check all that apply)
- ❏ Grady Memorial Hospital
- ❏ Good Samaritan
- ❏ Lakewood Health Center (Lakewood Avenue)
- ❏ South Fulton Medical Center (Carver High School Campus)
- ❏ South Fulton Medical Center (Cleveland Avenue)
- ❏ Southside Medical Center (Ridge Avenue)
- ❏ Atlanta Medical Piedmont
- ❏ Private physician (Please List Location) _____
- ❏ Urgent Care (Please List Location) _____
- ❏ Veterans Administration Hospital (VA)
- ❏ Nowhere, home remedies only
- ❏ Other (Please List) _____

23 How often do you usually get health care at the location(s) above?
- ❏ Annually
- ❏ Monthly
- ❏ Quarterly
- ❏ Weekly
- ❏ Other (Please specify):

24 What services/resources are available in your community? (Check all that apply)
- ❏ Community Clinic
- ❏ Counseling Services
- ❏ Home Health
- ❏ Hospital
- ❏ Private Clinic
- ❏ Urgent Care
- ❏ YMCA (or Other Community Center)
- ❏ Other (Please List) _____

NOW, WE WOULD LIKE TO KNOW THE BEST WAY TO SHARE HEALTH SERVICE AND RESOURCE INFORMATION WITH YOU

25 What are the **three** best ways to share health information **with you**? Please <u>rank your top</u> **three** <u>choices.</u> **(Write "1" next to the choice that is the best, "2" the second best, and "3" the third best way.)**

	Ranking
Attend Church Events	
Attend Community Events	
Email	
E-News Bulletin/E-Health Cards	
Facebook	
Flyers	
Health Clinics	
Health Fairs	
Instagram	
Internet	
Local Newspapers	
Neighborhood Meetings	
Phone	
Posters	
Radio Programs	
School Meetings	
Television Programs	
Twitter	
Word of Mouth	
Other (Please List)	
_____	

26 Please share any other ideas or comments about health concerns for you and your community.

NOW, WE WOULD LIKE TO KNOW ABOUT MORE ABOUT YOU

27 What is your age? (Check One)
○ 18–24 years
○ 25–34 years
○ 35–44 years
○ 45–54 years

○ 55–64 years
○ 65 years or older

28 What is your gender?
○ Male
○ Female
○ Transgender

29 Are you Hispanic or Latino?
○ Yes
○ No

30 What do you consider your race to be? (Check all that apply)
○ American Indian or Alaskan Native
○ Asian
○ Black/African American
○ Native-Hawaiian or Other Pacific Islander
○ White
○ Other (Please Specify) _____

31 Now thinking about your physical health, which includes physical illness and injury, for how many days during the past 30 days was your physical health not good?

32 Now thinking about your mental health, which includes stress, depression, and problems with emotions, for how many days during the past 30 days was your mental health not good?

33 Do you have a substance use issue?
○ Yes
○ No

34 What Neighborhood Planning Unit (NPU) do you **work** in?
○ I
○ V

○ X
○ Y
○ Z
○ Other (Please Specify) _____
○ Don't Know

35 What is your total family household income in a year?
○ Under $10,000
○ $10,001–$25,000
○ $25,001–$40,000
○ $40,001–$55,000
○ $55,001–$75,000
○ $75,001–$100,000
○ Over $100,000
○ I prefer not to disclose my income.

36 Please indicate your marital status.
○ Single, Never Married
○ Informally Married or Living with a Permanent Partner
○ Married
○ Divorced
○ Widowed
○ I prefer not to disclose this information.

37 Please indicate your sexual orientation.
○ Bisexual
○ Gay
○ Heterosexual
○ Lesbian
○ Other (please specify)
○ I prefer not to disclose this information.

38 Please tell us more about the children in your household (please check all that apply).
○ Reside with children under 6 years old
○ Reside with children 6 to 17 years old
○ No children under 18 years old in the household.
○ I prefer not to disclose this information.

39 Please indicate your household size.
○ 1-person household
○ 2-person household

○ 3-person household
○ 4-person household
○ 5-person household
○ 6-person household
○ 7-or-more-person household
○ I prefer not to disclose this information.

THANK YOU FOR TAKING TIME TO COMPLETE THIS SURVEY!

If you have any questions or concerns, please contact the Morehouse School of Medicine Prevention Research Center (MSM PRC) at 404-752-1022.

Morehouse School of Medicine Prevention Research Center. (2017). *Community Health Needs and Assets Assessment.* [Survey]

Windshield Survey

Date _____

Community Boundaries
North _____
South _____
East _____
West _____

Survey Time
Day   _____
Night _____

Description of Typical Housing:

Description of Recreational Outlets:

Description of Commercial Facilities:

Description of Social Activities:

Description of Building:

Description of Residents' Front Yards:

Tally of Abandoned Vehicles_____

Tally of Retail Stores_____

Number of Schools_____

Description of Areas Where People Congregate:

Number of Churches_____

Number of Liquor Stores_____

Number of Potholes_____

Is Street Light Adequate: Yes _____   No _____   Maybe _____

Description of Human Service Agencies:

Description of "Children at Play":

Name of Person(s) Conducting Survey
_____
_____

Was this a walking survey: Yes _____   No _____

Was this a driving survey: Yes _____   No _____

Start Time _____
End Time _____

Description of Area Covered:

Additional Information/Other:

Morehouse School of Medicine

Community Coalition Board (CCB) Satisfaction Survey Priority Areas and Sample Questions

1. **How long** have you been a member of the MSM PRC Community Coalition Board (CCB)?
○ A. Less than one year
○ B. 1 to 4 years
○ C. 5 or more

Please select the response that best shows how satisfied you are with each aspect of the CCB that is described. Your additional comments in each area are strongly encouraged to support improvement efforts.

Sample Questions	Very Dissatisfied	Dissatisfied	Neutral	Satisfied	Very Satisfied
Clarity of the vision for where the CCB is going					
Follow through on the CCB's activities					

Please select the response that best shows how satisfied you are with the **leadership.**

Sample Questions	Very Dissatisfied	Dissatisfied	Neutral	Satisfied	Very Satisfied
Opportunities for CCB members to take leadership roles in PRC initiatives					
CCB leadership's active engagement of CCB members					
Collaboration between MSM PRC staff/faculty and CCB members					

Please select the response that best shows how satisfied you are with the **involvement in the CCB.**

Sample Questions	Very Dissatisfied	Dissatisfied	Neutral	Satisfied	Very Satisfied
The CCB's collaboration(s) with local communities/ coalitions					
Collaborative activities among CCB members					

Please select the response that best shows how satisfied you are with the **communication.**

Sample Questions	Very Dissatisfied	Dissatisfied	Neutral	Satisfied	Very Satisfied
Use of communication tools to promote awareness of the CCB's goals, actions, and accomplishments					
Communication between and among CCB members and MSM PRC staff/ faculty					

Please select the response that best represents your opinion about **your work with the CCB.**

Sample Questions	Strongly Disagree	Disagree	Neutral	Agree	Strongly Agree
My abilities are used effectively					
My time is well spent on the CCB					

Please select the response that best represents your opinion about the CCB.

1. What are the top three areas in which the CCB excels?

2. What are the top three areas in which the CCB needs improvement?

3. What specific and practical steps do you recommend for CCB improvement?

Medical Student–Developed Surveys

Community Survey

Group I

1. _____Gender   2. _____Employment Status

__M __F   __Employed ___Retired __Unemployed

3. Marital Status

_____Single ___Married ___Divorced ____Widowed

4. Age   5. Registered to vote   6. Number of children under age 18 ____
__ 18–25   __Yes __No
__ 26–35
__ 36–45
__ 46–55
__ 56–65
__ 66+

7. Where do you receive most of your health care?
__ Grady Memorial Hospital
__ Southside Medical Center (Southside Healthcare)
__ Private doctor
__ Fulton County Department of Health and Wellness (Health Dept.)
__ South Fulton Medical Center (S. Fulton Hospital)
__ Center for Black Women's Wellness
__ Other (specify) _____

8. Do you have:
__ Private insurance (includes employment-based, individual policy, BC/BS,
    Aetna, etc.)
__ Medicaid
__ Medicare

__ None of the above
__ No answer, don't know

9. Do you have health insurance coverage for your children?
__ Yes   __ No   __ No children under 18 years old

10. In the past 12 months, how many times have you or your family members used the emergency room for your medical care?
__ Never   __ 1   __ 2   __ 3   __ 4   __ 5   __ >5

For each of the following questions, indicate whether you
SA—Strongly agree   A—Agree   N—Neutral   D—Disagree   SD—Strongly Disagree

____ 11. I can shop for most of my household supplies (such as groceries) in my community.
____ 12. I usually feel safe in my community.
____ 13. I get at least 30 minutes of exercise or physical activity 5 times a week or more.
____ 14. I eat at least 5 portions of fruits and vegetables every day.
____ 15. I am familiar with the Center for Working Families.
____ 16. This community has adequate recreational activities for youth.
____ 17. Renovations and development in this community have been very beneficial.
____ 18. I generally feel upbeat and hopeful about life.

19. How would you rate your own health?
__ Excellent
__ Good
__ Fair
__ Poor

20. What do you think is the most important health problem in this community?
__ Heart disease
. Cancer
__ High blood pressure
__ Diabetes
__ Mental health
__ Teen pregnancy
__ Drug abuse
__ Sexually transmitted diseases and AIDS
__ Other (Specify) _____

21. Other than health problems, what do you think is the most important problem in this community?
___ Unemployment
___ Crime and violence
___ Lack of after-school programs or other recreational activities for youth
___ Lack of role models for youth
___ Deteriorating housing
___ Trash and junk
___ Other (Specify) _____

22. Which of the following programs would be most helpful to you or to your family?
___ Health education for adults (for instance, covering nutrition, exercise, healthy living, etc.)
___ Health education or life skills training for youth (covering drugs, tobacco, sex, exercise, etc.)
___ After-school program for kids, including exercise (sports) and help with homework
___ Job training
___ Smoking cessation
___ Financial counseling
___ Drug or alcohol counseling and treatment

21. What group of people in your community needs additional support or additional services?
___ School age children (8–18 years)
___ Young adults (18–25 years)
___ Single parents
___ Men
___ Women
___ Seniors (55+years)
___ Other (specify) _____

22. Community: ___ Mechanicsville ___ Peoplestown ___ Pittsburgh ___ Cap Sumhill ___

NUTRITION SURVEY

- What fruits and vegetables do you want us to offer?

o Oranges	o Mustard greens
o Grapes	o Collard greens
o Apples	o Green beans
o Pears	o Broccoli
o Grapefruit	o Cabbage
o Other_____	o Other_____

- Where do you normally buy fruits and vegetables?
  - o Shoppers Market ("Korean Store")   o Kroger   o Other_____

- Have you ever purchased fruits or vegetables from us before? ___Yes ___No

- How did you hear about us?

- How many children do you have who are 0–5 years old___ 6–11 years old___ over 11 years old___?

- How many children do you have who are students at Tull Waters School? ___

- About how many servings of fruits & vegetables do you eat per day? ___

- How many servings of fruits and vegetables do you think you <u>should</u> eat per day? ___

- What foods are high in (check 2 in each category):
  - Vitamin C?
    - ___Oranges
    - ___Broccoli
    - ___Peanuts
  - Iron?
    - ___Spinach
    - ___Potatoes
    - ___Turnip greens
  - Fiber?
    - Cheese
    - ___Apples
    - ___Beans

Faculty Community Engagement List of Publications

Akintobi, T. H., et al. 2016. "Applying a Community-Based Participatory Research Approach to Address Determinants of Cardiovascular Disease and Diabetes Mellitus in an Urban Setting." In *Handbook of Community-Based Participatory Research*, ed. S. Coughlin, S. Smith, and M. Fernandez, 131–54. New York: Oxford University Press.

Akintobi, T. H., et al. 2018. "Processes and Outcomes of a Community-Based Participatory Research-Driven Health Needs Assessment: A Tool for Moving Health Disparity Research to Action." *Progress in Community Health Partnerships* 12 (1S): 139–47.

Akintobi, T. H., J. C. Trotter, D. Evans, T. Johnson, N. Laster, D. Jacobs, and T. King. 2011. "Applications in Bridging the Gap: A Community-Campus Partnership to Address Sexual Health Disparities among African-American Youth in the South." *Journal of Community Health* 36:486–94.

Alema-Mensah, E., S. A. Smith, M. Claridy, V. Ede, B. Ansa, and D. S. Blumenthal. 2017. "Social Networks as Predictors of Colorectal Cancer Screening in African Americans." *Journal of the Georgia Public Health Association* 6 (3): 369–72.

Apantaku-Onayemi, F., W. Baldyga, S. Amuwo, A. Adefuye, T. Mason, R. Mitchell, and D. S. Blumenthal. 2012. "Driving to Better Health: Cancer and Cardiovascular Risk Assessment among Taxicab Drivers in Chicago." *Journal of Health Care for the Poor and Underserved* 23:768–80.

Bacquet, C., and R. Braithwaite. 2009. "Health Disparity (HD) Issues That Affect Underserved and Racially or Ethnically Diverse Communities, Including African American, Underserved and Samoan Communities." *Journal of Health Care for the Poor and Underserved* 20 (2 Suppl.): 1–2.

Belloni, J. S., et al. 1991. "Application of Principles of Community Intervention." *Public Health Reports* 106 (3): 244–47.

Blumenthal, D. S. 1978. "Building a Base for Reform." *Southern Exposure* 6 (2): 83–89.

Blumenthal, D. S. 1990. "The Area Health Education Center Model of Community-Based Health Sciences Education." *Annals of Community-Oriented Education* 3:85–90.

Blumenthal, D. S. 2002. "Community Service and Social Justice." *Brookings Review* 20 (4): 25–26.

Blumenthal, D. S. 2006. "A Community Coalition Board Creates a Set of Values for Community-Based Research." *Preventing Chronic Disease* [serial online]. http://www.cdc.gov/pcd/issues/2006/jan/05_0068.htm.

Blumenthal, D. S. 2006. "Community Outreach at Morehouse School of Medicine." *Atlanta Medicine* 79 (1): 9–13.

Blumenthal, D. S. 2011. "Is Community-Based Participatory Research Possible?" *American Journal of Preventive Medicine* 40:386–89.

Blumenthal, D. S. 2013. "Academic-Community Partnerships for CEOD." In *Community Engagement, Organization, and Development for Public Health Practice*, ed. F. G. Murphy, 117–30. New York: Springer.

Blumenthal, D. S., R. DiClemente, R. L. Braithwaite, and S. Smith, eds. 2013. *Community-Based Participatory Research: Issues, Methods, and Translation to Practice*. 2nd ed. New York: Springer.

Blumenthal, D. S., J. Fort, N. U. Ahmed, K. A. Semenya, G. B. Schreiber, S. Perry, and J. Guillory. 2005. "Impact of a Two-City Community Cancer Prevention Intervention on African-Americans." *Journal of the National Medical Association* 97:1479–88.

Blumenthal, D. S., S. A. Smith, C. D. Majett, and E. Alema-Mensah. 2010. "A Trial of Three Interventions to Promote Colorectal Cancer Screening in African Americans." *Cancer* 116:922–29.

Blumenthal, D. S., J. Sung, J. Williams, J. Liff, and R. Coates. 1995. "Recruitment and Retention of Subjects for a Longitudinal Cancer Prevention Study in an Inner-City Black Community." *Health Services Research* 30:197–205.

Bolar, C., N. Hernandez, T. H. Akintobi, C. McAllister, A. Ferguson, L. Rollins, G. Wrenn, M. Okafor, D. Collins, and T. Clem. 2016. "Context Matters: A Community-Based Study of Urban Minority Parents' Views on Child Health." *Journal of the Georgia Public Health Association* 5 (3): 212–19.

Braithwaite, R. L. 1992. "Coalition Partnerships for Health Promotion and Empowerment." In *Health Issues in the Black Community*, ed. R. Braithwaite and S. Taylor, 321–37. San Francisco: Jossey-Bass.

Braithwaite, R. L. 1994. "Challenges to Evaluation in Rural Coalitions." *Journal of Community Psychology*, Special Issue, 188–200.

Braithwaite, R. L., J. Austin, and S. F. Taylor. 1999. "Building Health Coalitions in Black Communities." Newbury Park, CA: Sage.

Braithwaite, R. L., C. Bianchi, and S. E. Taylor. 1994. "An Ethnographic Approach to Community Organization and Health Empowerment." *Health Education Quarterly* 21 (3): 407–16.

Braithwaite, R. L., and N. Lythcott. 1989. "Community Empowerment as a Strategy for Health Promotion for Black and Other Minorities." *Journal of the American Medical Association* 261 (2): 282–83.

Braithwaite, R. L., F. Murphy, N. Lythcott, and D. Blumenthal. 1989. "Community Organization and Development for Health Promotion within an Urban Black Community: A Conceptual Model." *Health Education* 20 (5): 56–60.

Braithwaite, R., M. Ro, K. Braithwaite, and H. Treadwell. 2006. "Community Voices: Health Care for the Underserved." *Journal of Health Care for the Poor and Underserved* 17 (1 Suppl.).

Braithwaite, R. L. 1998. "Culturally Based Health Promotion: Practices and Systems." *Cultural Competence for Health Care Professionals Working with African-American Communities: Theory and Practice*. Cultural Competence Series #7, HRSA, DHHS Publication No. (SMA) 98-3238.

Braithwaite, R. L. 1991. Review of *Terms of Empowerment: The Consumer's Guide To Medical Lingo*, by Charles Inlander and Paula Brisco. *Journal of Health Care for the Poor and Underserved* 1 (4): 424–26.

Braithwaite, R. L. 2000. "Definition of Empowerment." *Encyclopedia of Psychology*. American Psychological Association.

Braithwaite, R. L., and R. McKenzie. 2012. "The Utility of Large Coalitions for Community Health Programs." *Journal of Health Care for the Poor and Underserved* 23:4–6.

Braithwaite, R. L., R. McKenzie, V. Pruitt, K. B. Holden, K. Aaron, and C. Hollimon. 2012. "Community-Based Participatory Evaluation: The Healthy Start Approach." *Journal of Health Promotion Practice* 13:2.

Braun, K. L., et al. 2012. "Operationalization of Community-Based Participatory Research Principles: Assessment of the National Cancer Institute's Community Network Programs." *American Journal of Public Health* 102 (6): 1195–203.

Braun, K. L., et al. 2015. "The National Cancer Institute's Community Networks Program Initiative to Reduce Cancer Health Disparities: Outcomes and Lessons Learned." *Progress in Community Health Partnerships: Research, Education, and Action* 9:21–32.

Caplan, L., T. H. Akintobi, T. Gordon, T. Zellner, S. Smith, and D. Blumenthal. 2016. "Reducing Disparities by Way of a Cancer Disparities Research Training Program." *Journal of Health Disparities Research and Practice* 9 (3): 103–14.

Erwin, K., D. S. Blumenthal, T. Chapel, and L. V. Allwood. 2004. "Building an Academic-Community Partnership for Increasing the Representation of Minorities in the Health Professions." *Journal of Health Care for the Poor and Underserved* 15:589–602.

Estape, E. S., M. H. Mays, R. Harrigan, and R. Mayberry. 2014. "Incorporating Translational Research with Clinical Research to Increase Effectiveness in Healthcare for Better Health." *Clinical and Translational Medicine* 3:20.

Gaglioti, A., X. Junjun, L. Rollins, P. Baltrus, K. O'Connell, D. Cooper, J. Hopkins, N. Botchwey, and T. H. Akintobi. 2018. "Neighborhood Environmental Health and Premature Cardiovascular Death in Atlanta: A Secondary Data Analysis Motivated by Community Wisdom from the REACH Project." *Preventing Chronic Disease* 15:E17. doi:10.5888/pcd15.170220.

Henry Akintobi, T., R. Braithwaite, and A. Dodds. 2014. "Residential Segregation—Trends and Implications for Conducting Effective Community-Based Research to Address Ethnic Health Disparities." In *Uprooting Urban America: Multidisciplinary Perspectives on Race, Class and Gentrification*, ed. H. Hall, C. Cole-Robinson, and A. Kohli, 157–69. New York: Peter Lang.

Henry Akintobi, T., N. Dawood, and D. Blumenthal. 2014. "An Academic-Public Health Department Partnership for Education, Research, Practice and Governance." *Journal of Public Health Management and Practice* 20 (3): 310–14.

Henry Akintobi, T., et al. 2018. "Processes and Outcomes of a Community-Based Participatory Research-Driven Health Needs Assessment: A Tool for Moving Health Disparity Reporting to Evidence-Based Action." *Progress in Community Health Partnerships: Research, Education, and Action* 12 (1S): 139–47.

Henry Akintobi, T., D. Evans Wilkerson, K. Rodgers, C. Escoffery, R. Haardörfer, and M. Kegler. 2016. "Assessment of the Building Collaborative Research Capacity Model: Bridging the Community-Academic Researcher Divide." *Journal of the Georgia Public Health Association* 6 (2): 123–32.

Henry Akintobi, T., L. Goodin, and L. Hoffman. 2013. "Morehouse School of Medicine Prevention Research Center: Collaborating with Neighborhoods to Develop Community-Based Participatory Approaches to Address Health Disparities in Metropolitan Atlanta." *Atlanta Medicine: Journal of the Medical Association of Atlanta* 84 (2): 14–17.

Henry Akintobi, T., L. Goodin, E. Trammel, D. Collins, and D. Blumenthal. 2011. "How Do You Set Up and Maintain a Community Advisory Board?" (Chapter 5, Section 4b, 136–38) of "Challenges in Improving Community Engaged Research," Clinical and Translational Science Award Community Engagement Key Function Committee Task Force on the Principles of Community Engagement, *Principles of Community Engagement*, 2nd ed. Washington, DC: US Department of Health and Human Services.

Henry Akintobi, T., L. Hoffman, C. McAllister, L. Goodin, N. Hernandez, L. Rollins, and A. Miller. 2016. "Assessing the Oral Health Needs of Black Men in Low-Income, Urban Communities." *American Journal of Men's Health* 12 (2): 326–37.

Henry Akintobi, T., J. Trotter, D. Evans, N. Laster, and T. Johnson. 2013. "Community-Based Participatory Approaches to Evaluation." In *Community-Based Participatory Health Research*, 2nd ed., ed. D. Blumenthal, R. Braithwaite, and S. Smith, 231–62. New York: Springer.

Henry Akintobi, T., E. Yancey, R. Mayberry, P. Daniels, D. Jacobs, and J. Berry. 2012. "Using Evaluability Assessment and Valuation Capacity Building to Strengthen Community-Based HIV/AIDS Prevention Initiatives in the South." *Journal of Health Care for the Poor and Underserved* 23 (2): 33–48.

Henry Akintobi, T., E. Yancey, D. Muteteke, and J. Bailey. 2004. "Partnership for Evaluation of the Bilingual Bicultural Service Demonstration Program: Merging Public Health Research and Practice." *Journal of Interprofessional Care* 18 (4): 440–41.

Hoffman, L. M., L. Rollins, T. H. Akintobi, C. McAllister, N. Hernandez, K. Erwin, and A. Miller. 2017. "Evaluation of a Community-Based Participatory Oral Health Intervention for Low-Income African American Men." *American Journal of Public Health* 107 (S1): 104–10.

Holden, K., B. McGregor, A. Belton, J. Hopkins, S. Blanks, and G. Wrenn. 2016. "Community Engaged Leadership to Advance Health Equity and Build Healthier Communities." *Social Sciences* 5 (1): 2. doi:10.3390/socsci5010002.

Josiah Willock, R., R. M. Mayberry, F. Yan, and P. Daniels. 2015. "Peer Training of Community Health Workers to Improve Heart Health among African American Women." *Health Promotion Practice* 16 (1): 63–71.

Irwin, C., and R. L. Braithwaite. 1997. "A Church-Based Diabetes Education Program for Older, African-American Women." *American Journal of Health Studies* 13 (1): 1–7.

Kegler, M. C., D. S. Blumenthal, T. H. Akintobi, K. Rodgers, K. Erwin, W. Thompson, and E. Hopkins. 2016. "Lessons Learned from Three Models That Use Small

Grants for Building Academic-Community Partnerships for Research." *Journal of Health Care for the Poor and Underserved* 27 (2): 527–48.

Langley, W. M., and W. Kahnweiler. 2003. "The Role of Pastoral Leadership in the Sociopolitically Active African American Church," *Organizational Development Journal* 21 (2): 43–51.

Mayberry, R., R. Josiah Willock, and P. V. Daniels. 2012. "Community Capacity Building and Community Health Workers." In *Community Engagement, Organization and Development for Public Health Practice*, ed. F. Murphy. New York: Springer.

Mayberry, R. M., P. Daniels, A. Bazzell, F. Yan, R. Josiah Willock, and B. Mack. 2013. "Survey Planning and Implementation in the Context of CBPR." In *Community-Based Participatory Health Research: Issues, Methods, and Translation to Practice*, 2nd ed., ed. D. S. Blumenthal, R. J. DiClemente, R. L. Braithwaithe, and S. A. Smith. New York: Springer.

Mayberry, R. M., P. Daniels, T. Henry Akintobi, E. M. Yancey, J. Berry, and N. Clark. 2008. "Community-Based Organizations' Capacity to Plan, Implement, and Evaluate Success." *Journal of Community Health* 33 (5): 285–92.

Mayberry, R. M., P. Daniels, T. Henry Akintobi, E. M. Yancey, J. Berry, and N. Clark. 2009. "Enhancing Community-Based Organizations' Capacity for HIV/AIDS Education and Prevention." *Evaluation and Program Planning* 32 (3): 213–20.

Neighbors, H. W., R. L. Braithwaite, and E. Thompson. 1995. "Health Promotion and African-Americans: From Personal Empowerment to Community Action." *American Journal of Health Promotion* 9 (4): 281–87.

Quinn, G., T. Albrecht, R. Marshall, and T. Henry Akintobi. 2005. "Thinking Like a Marketer: Training for a Shift in the Mindset of the Public Health Workforce." *Health Promotion Practice* 6 (2): 157–63.

Reese, L., D. S. Blumenthal, and V. Haynes. 2012. "The Southeastern U.S. Collaborative Center of Excellence for the Elimination of Disparities (SUCCEED): Reducing Breast and Cervical Cancer Disparities for African American Women." *Journal of Health Care for the Poor and Underserved* 23:49–61.

Rogers, K., T. Akintobi, W. Thompson, C. Escoffery, D. Evans, and M. Kegler. 2014. "A Model for Strengthening Collaborative Research Capacity: Illustrations from the Atlanta Clinical Translational Science Institute." *Health Education and Behavior* 41 (3): 267–74.

Rollins, L., T. Akintobi, A. Hermstad, D. Cooper, L. Goodin, J. Beane, S. Spivey, A. Riedesel, L. Taylor, and R. Lyn. 2017. "Community-Based Approaches to Reduce Chronic Disease Disparities in Georgia." *Journal of the Georgia Public Health Association* 6 (4): 402–10.

Rollins, L., A. Sy, N. Crowell, D. Rivers, A. Miller, P. Cooper, D. Teague, C. Jackson, T. Henry Akintobi, and E. Ofili. 2018. "Learning and Action in Community Health: Using the Health Belief Model to Assess and Educate African American Community Residents about Participation in Clinical Research." *International Journal of Environmental Research and Public Health* 15 (9): 1862.

Satcher, D. 2006. "Working in and with Communities to Eliminate Disparities in Health." *Health Promotion Practice* 7 (3 Suppl.): S176-78.

Satcher, D. 2011. "Pioneers in Health Equity: Lessons from the REACH Communities." *Minority Health Archives*.

Smith, S., L. Johnson, D. Wesley, K. B. Turner, G. McCray, J. Sheats, and D. Blumenthal. 2012. "Translation to Practice of an Intervention to Promote Colorectal Cancer Screening among African Americans." *Clinical and Translational Science* 5:412–15.

Smith, S. A., E. Alema-Mensah, W. Yoo, B. Ansa, and D. S. Blumenthal. 2017. "Persons Who Failed to Obtain Colorectal Cancer Screening Despite Participation in an Evidence-Based Intervention." *Journal of Community Health* 42 (1): 30–34.

Smith, S. A., and D. S. Blumenthal. 2012. "Community Health Workers Support Community-Based Participatory Research Ethics: Lessons Learned along the Research-to-Practice-to-Community Continuum." *Journal of Health Care for the Poor and Underserved* 23 (4 Suppl.): 77–87.

Smith, S. A., M. S. Whitehead, J. Q. Sheats, B. E. Ansa, S. S. Coughlin, and D. S. Blumenthal. 2015. "Community-Based Participatory Research Principles for the African American Community." *Journal of the Georgia Public Health Association* 5:52–56.

Sufian, M., J. Grunbaum, T. Akintobi, A. Dozier, M. Eder, S. Jones, P. Mullan, C. R. Weir, and S. White-Cooper. 2011. "Program Evaluation and Evaluating Community Engagement" (163–82). Clinical and Translational Science Award Community Engagement Key Function Committee Task Force on the Principles of Community Engagement. *Principles of Community Engagement*, 2nd ed. Washington, DC: US Department of Health and Human Services.

Sung, J., D. S. Blumenthal, R. J. Coates, J. Williams, E. Alema-Mensah, and J. M. Liff. 1997. "Effect of a Cancer Screening Intervention Conducted by Lay Health Workers among Inner-City Women." *American Journal of Preventive Medicine* 13:51–57.

Taylor, C., M. Langley, and J. Leonard. 2010. "Church-Based Health Promotion to Address Chronic Diseases among African Americans." In *Diabetes in Black American: Public Health and Clinical Solutions to a National Crisis*, ed. Jack Leonard Jr. Crown Point, IN: Hilton.

Treadwell, H. M., B. J. Sabol, K. B. Holden, and R. L. Braithwaite. 2010. "Conclusion: When the Community Voices Initiative Began, We Did Not Know What We Did Not Know . . ." In *Community Voices Health Matters*, 301–20. San Francisco: Jossey-Bass.

Wallerstein, N., et al. (1994). "Community Empowerment Forum." *Health Education Quarterly* 21 (3): 281–94.

Wingfield, J., T. Henry Akintobi, D. Jacobs, and M. Ford. 2012. "The SUCCEED Legacy Grant Program: Enhancing Community Capacity to Implement Evidence-Based Interventions in Breast and Cervical Cancer." *Journal of Health Care for the Poor and Underserved* 23 (2): 62–76.

for, 61, 102; and research partner communities, 62; research priorities of, 64

primary care, 31; as medical school curriculum track, 42; MSM's commitment to, 40, 90, 101–2

primary care physicians: as priority health concern, 31, 38, 183, 190

problem identification: as aspect of the Morehouse Model, 7–8

project development: as aspect of the Morehouse Model, 11–12

PROMETRA (Promocion de la Medicina Tradicional Amazonica), 53

public health: definitions of, 49; and social accountability, 49–53. *See also* master of public health program at MSM

Quinnipiac University (CT) Netter School of Medicine, 190

Racial and Ethnic Approaches to Community Health (REACH), 156–57

recognition: as aspect of the Morehouse Model, 15–16

Report of the Graduate Medical Education National Advisory Committee (GMENAC), 180–81, 183

research: as aspect of medical education, 196–98; and community leadership, 166–67; and social accountability, 47–48; translational, 78–80, 100, 162, 169–70, 197–98. *See also* community-based participatory research; Prevention Research Center; Medical Student Summer Research Experience

Research!America, 196–97

research partner communities (RPCs): and the Prevention Research Center, 62, 69, 70

Rice, Valerie Montgomery, 118, 170

rural communities: case studies involving, 126, 133–46; challenges of working with, 129–33; community engagement in, 124, 126–33, 146–47; defining, 124–26; distrust of outsiders in, 129; health disparities in, 121–22,

130; health promotion in, 93, 122–24, 165; life expectancy in, 121; as part of medical school curriculum, 193; training for, 95

Rural Health Clerkship: as part of MSM curriculum, 45

Satcher Health Leadership Institute (SHLI), 167–69

sex education: in rural communities, 133–36

sexually transmitted diseases (STDs), 71; in rural communities, 137–40

Simmons, Henry, 115–16

simulations: as used in medical education, 184–85

Smart and Secure Children (SSC) Program, 155–56, 167–68

social accountability of medical schools, 29–32, 199; awards for, 35; criteria for assessment of, 33–37, 54–55; definitions of, 30, 33; and health promotion services, 49; and international engagement, 53–54; literature on, 31; and MSM, 31–32, 37–47, 54–55; principles and values associated with, 34–35; and public health, 49–53; and research, 47–48

social determinants: of health, 45, 63, 68, 91, 118, 121, 122

social justice: and the role of coalitions, 113–14

social mission, 31, 36, 101. *See also* social accountability

Social Mission Metrics Initiative, 37

Southeastern Primary Care Consortium, 99

Southeastern US Collaborative Center of Excellence in the Elimination of Health Disparities (SUCCEED), 97

Southern Illinois University, 186–87

standardized patients: as used in medical education, 184–85

Stellenbosch University, 53

Still School of Osteopathic Medicine, 193

Strategic Prevention Framework (SPF): and the Health Promotion Resource Center, 141, 142, 145–46